Becoming a Trainer in Adult Abuse Work

of related interest

Elder Abuse Work
Best Practice in Britain and Canada
Edited by Jacki Pritchard
ISBN 1 85302 704 9

Working with Elder Abuse
A Training Manual for Home Care, Residential and Day Care Staff
Jacki Pritchard
ISBN 1 85302 418 X

The Abuse of Older People
A Training Manual for Detection and Prevention, 2nd edition
Jacki Pritchard
ISBN 1 85302 305 1

Geronticide
Killing the Elderly
Mike Brogden
ISBN 1 85302 709 X

Care Services for Later Life
Transformations and Critiques
Edited by Tony Warnes, Lorna Warren and Mike Nolan
ISBN 1 85302 852 5

Past Trauma in Late Life
European Perspectives on Therapeutic Work with Older People
Edited by Linda Hunt, Mary Marshall and Cherry Rowlings
ISBN 1 85302 446 5

Understanding Dementia
The Man with the Worried Eyes
Richard Cheston and Michael Bender
ISBN 1 85302 479 1

Training and Development for Dementia Care Workers
Anthea Innes
ISBN 1 85302 761 8

Including the Person with Dementia in Designing and Delivering Care
'I Need to Be Me!'
Elizabeth Barnett
Foreword by Mary Marshall
ISBN 1 85302 740 5

Social Work and Dementia
Good Practice and Care Management
Margaret Anne Tibbs
Foreword by Murna Downs
ISBN 1 85302 904 1

Becoming a Trainer in Adult Abuse Work

A Practical Guide

Jacki Pritchard

Jessica Kingsley Publishers
London and Philadelphia

First published in the United Kingdom in 2001 by
Jessica Kingsley Publishers Ltd,
116 Pentonville Road, London
N1 9JB, England

and

325 Chestnut Street,
Philadelphia PA 19106, USA.

www.jkp.com

© Copyright 2001 Jacki Pritchard

Library of Congress Cataloging in Publication Data

A CIP catalog record for this book is available from the Library of Congress

British Library Cataloguing in Publication Data

A CIP catalogue record for this book is available from the British Library

ISBN 1 85302 913 0

Printed and Bound in Great Britain by
Athenaeum Press, Gateshead, Tyne and Wear

Contents

The following symbols have been used throughout the book for ease of recognition:

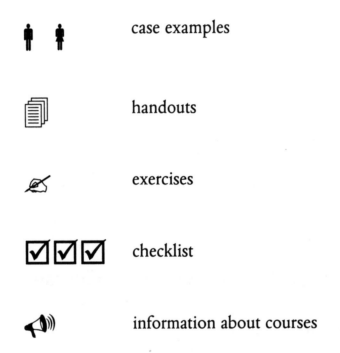

case examples

handouts

exercises

checklist

information about courses

All pages marked ✓ may be photocopied for training pages, but may not be reproduced in other forms without the prior permission of the publisher.

For Eric and Audrey Sainsbury, who are always there for me

Acknowledgments

I would like to thank all the people I have trained over the past 13 years and also the numerous organisations who have brought me in to train their staff. Without them I would not have gained the experience to write this guide. I would also like to thank Mary Shimwell, who was the first person ever to ask me to provide training, which was to a group of nurses.

Catherine Sawdon has also played a crucial part in my own professional development; in the early years she shared so much of her knowledge and experience with me about adult learning, practice teaching and training.

I am totally indebted to Zetta Bear and Ron Wiener, who have taught me so much over the years and continue to be great sources of knowledge, wisdom and support.

I am grateful to the organisations that have allowed me to use their materials as examples of good practice in this guide; in particular Wakefield Housing and Social Care, Wakefield Metropolitan District Council and the City of Stoke of Trent Social Services Department.

Glossary of Terms

Adult abuse work   This includes prevention, investigation and intervention in working with adults who are the victims of abuse (physical, emotional, financial, neglect and sexual).

Leader   Person who is going to train the trainers in a pool.

Organisation   This includes organisations within any sector (statutory, voluntary, independent) that could be involved in adult abuse work.

Participant   Person on a training course (including those on training-the-trainers courses).

Pool   Workers who have been brought together to provide training on adult abuse.

Trainer   Person who provides training. This could be someone within a training section, in a pool or an independent trainer.

Training officer   This includes anyone who has responsibility for organising training within an organisation or specific work setting, e.g. staff within traditional training sections; deputy managers in residential settings; development officers with a responsibility for training in adult abuse.

Worker   Person at any level working in any setting/organisation within the statutory, voluntary or independent sectors.

Introduction

I have been training on the subject of abuse (both child and adult) for the past 13 years and have learnt many painful lessons during the course of that time. When I started training I was working as a generic social worker, but at the same time was undertaking research into elder abuse. Since then I have trained thousands of workers from all disciplines and sectors. For the past five years I have become more involved in training groups of practitioners who have been going to form pools of trainers on adult abuse within various organisations. I have found this work very challenging and exciting, but once again it has taught me many new lessons.

Sessions with potential trainers always remind me just how much you have to experience and then learn in order to become an effective trainer. If you have been training for a long time, you tend to take a lot for granted and forget how difficult it was at the outset. Reflecting on this recently has made me feel the time has come to write a short training guide to help people who may be starting out on this learning curve. I want to be able to share my own learning experiences with as many people as possible; writing a guide seemed the best way to achieve this.

Why now?

This guide is intended to address the issue of training on adult abuse work. I feel this is a critical time to be writing such a text. Most of this guide had been written before March 2000 when *No Secrets: Guidance on developing and implementing multi-agency policies and procedures to protect vulnerable adults from abuse* was launched by the Department of Health and Home Office (DOH 2000). Regarding training for staff and volunteers the guidance states:

5.2 Agencies should provide training for staff and volunteers on the policy, procedures and professional practices that are in place locally, commensurate with their responsibilities in the adult protection process. This should include:

- basic induction training with respect to awareness that abuse can take place and duty to report;

- more detailed awareness training, including training on recognition of abuse and responsibilities with respect to the procedures in their particular agency;

- specialist training for investigators; and

- specialist training for managers.

5.3 Training should take place at all levels in an organisation and within specified time scales. To ensure that procedures are carried out consistently no staff group should be excluded. Training should include issues relating to staff safety within a Health and Safety framework. Training is a continuing responsibility and should be provided as a rolling programme. (Unit Z1 of the NVQ Training Programme is specifically aimed at care workers in the community.) (page 23, DOH 2000)

This guidance does not tell me anything new. For years I have said that training should be ongoing for *all* staff. I have felt for a long time that certain groups are often omitted from training and that was my reason for writing a training manual especially for home care, residential and day care staff some years ago:

What has become painfully clear to me is that home care staff and staff working in residential units and day centres are crucial people in identifying abuse… Unfortunately, it is these two groups of staff who may not be seen as a priority for training in this area of work. Also, when they report suspected abuse they are often not listened to, not taken seriously, or ignored completely (because 'what do they know? They are not professionals'!) (page 1, Pritchard 1996)

But it is not just these two groups of staff who are often forgotten and not invited to inter-agency training. People forget local authority solicitors, housing officers, workers in housing associations, supported accommodation projects in the voluntary sector, volunteers, advocates and the list goes on. It is to be hoped that *No Secrets* will have an impact in the forthcoming years to improve the current situation.

The subject of adult abuse has gained recognition in the last decade but there are still insufficient resources being put into supporting practitioners who are working with abused people and their perpetrators. One of the reasons for this is that adult abuse work is still not statutory work and therefore is not given the same priority as child protection work. Consequently, the vast sums of money that are needed are not made readily available.

It is not my intention to present a negative picture here; we *have* made progress. I do not intend to present a summary of the historical developments in adult abuse work – that is not the purpose of this guide; there are many texts which address this elsewhere. However, it is important to explain that many organisations in the different sectors (statutory, voluntary and independent) now recognise that adult abuse is prevalent and must be addressed. Part of this task involves training the staff who are working with victims and abusers.

Over the years I have seen the development of elder abuse then adult abuse policies and procedures and have been involved in many working parties set up to write or review guidance. Resulting from those developments I have seen how different organisations have developed (or not developed) comprehensive training programmes for their staff. As I travel around the UK I have obtained a useful insight and it is quite horrifying to see the vast differences that exist. Some organisations put a great deal of effort into careful planning and then developing training programmes. Others just put on token courses on an ad hoc basis and there is no systematic scheme to support staff development in this subject area.

As I have already said, I have been involved in training pools of trainers for various organisations in the statutory, voluntary and independent sectors. I believe developing such pools is going to be the way forward and this is yet another reason for writing this guide now. I wanted to share my own learning experiences and pre-empt some of the questions and considerations which will face organisations and the staff who will have to take the lead in developing such pools.

Why pools of trainers?

It is generally accepted that to promote good practice in working with adult abuse we have to adopt the multi-disciplinary approach, in a similar way we do with child protection work. The reality is that this is extremely difficult to organise for a number of reasons that I shall now discuss.

In the early days of working with elder abuse (1980s) some social services departments developed their own policy and procedures and it was only later that other agencies signed up to the document. Even now, when policies are being rewritten, it is difficult to know how to extend the invitation to be involved in a working group. How far do you send draft documents out for consultation? There can also be conflict where perhaps an organisation has its own procedures. In my own experience I have known of NHS Trusts who have refused to be involved with the local adult-abuse working group and consequently refused to sign up to the final document. *No Secrets* does encourage inter-agency working by the formation of multi-agency management committees and mentions the issue of training:

> 3.4 To achieve effective inter-agency working, agencies may consider that there are merits in establishing a multi-agency management committee (adult protection), which is a standing committee of lead officers. Such a body should have a clearly defined remit and lines of accountability, and it should identify agreed objectives and priorities for its work. Such committees should determine policy, co-ordinate activity between agencies, facilitate joint training, and monitor and review progress. (page 15, DOH 2000)

Even if agencies do sign up to the final document, another problem then arises. How do you train the vast number of staff within all the agencies? Who should take the lead in organising this? Who bears the cost? It is not good enough for other agencies to rely on social services departments to take the lead in organising training programmes and then expect invitations for staff from other agencies to attend. Neither can one expect agencies to work on an individual basis i.e. with each agency developing their own training programme. There needs to be consistency in the way staff in all agencies are trained. Developing a pool of trainers is one way of addressing some of these problems.

Objectives of this guide

This guide is not going to give anyone *all* the answers on how to develop effective training. What I want it to do is to save people some time by raising issues they may not have thought of previously, point them in the right direction for information and training materials, and help them to avoid making some of the mistakes I have made myself.

The guide can be used by:

- organisations who are thinking about developing training programmes related to adult abuse

- training officers or other people who have lead responsibility for developing such programmes

- people who are responsible for co-ordinating National Vocational Qualification (NVQ) programmes

- practitioners who are thinking about becoming a trainer within a pool (or who have already volunteered) in any sector

- practitioners who are thinking about becoming independent trainers

- managers who need to train their staff group.

What the guide is and isn't

This guide is aimed at organisations and individuals who are starting to develop programmes and will be delivering basic awareness training. Its main objective is to help practitioners who are about to become trainers. It will *not* address delivering more advanced training courses. I believe very strongly that for more advanced and in-depth courses the trainer does need to have specific expertise in this area of work, i.e. s/he needs to have had direct experience of working with abuse. It is not enough to be able to present the academic perspective alone. I shall develop this discussion further in Chapters 1 and 5 and make suggestions as to the development of such programmes.

I need to emphasise again that this guide is a basic starting point. I wanted it to be a simple, helpful, realistic aid for people who do not have much time. It is not meant to be an academic text which includes loads of theory (e.g. about adult learning). I include a suggested reading list at the end so people can go in the right direction if they need to explore further. My intention is to save busy people time; the guide is meant to be a practical resource. I also hope that people will learn from my mistakes and that I pre-empt questions which are frequently asked when training the trainers.

Layout of the guide

I have tried to make this guide user-friendly by dividing it into chapters which will be easily accessible to people who have different needs. Chapters 1, 2 and 3 consider the development of training programmes on adult abuse within organisations, the selection of trainers and how to train and support those people. Chapters 4 and 5 go into specific detail about preparing for a training course and developing its contents. Chapters 6 and 7 look at the difficult issues and specific problems which a trainer may have to face; it is these areas that cause the most fear for inexperienced trainers. Chapter 8 discusses the importance of evaluation both for the organisation and the trainer. Case studies in Chapter 9 present materials which could be used in a basic awareness training course.

Throughout the guide there are references to other materials. I have chosen to include some materials from my other works that people have told me they have found particularly useful for workers in all sectors who work with vulnerable adults (not just older people) and would suggest that this guide be used in conjunction with those texts (Pritchard 1995 and 1996). A suggested reading list is presented at the end of the guide.

Terminology

A glossary is included (see page 9) so that the reader is clear about my use of terminology. I am very conscious of the fact that jargon within organisations can be confusing, and also this manual is likely to be used abroad.

I also want to explain why I choose to use the term 'adult abuse work' rather than 'adult protection work'. In my day-to-day work I think it is important to use the word 'abuse' in order to make people aware that adults *are* abused. It is a harsh reality and one about which we need to continually raise awareness. Sometimes abuse is minimised. There was a time in the early 1990s when people were advocating use of the term 'mistreatment' rather than 'abuse'. The word 'abuse' does make people feel uncomfortable, but abuse does happen and that is the reality we have to face. We should not get into avoidance!

I am not minimising the importance of protection work; it is of paramount importance. Any worker's prime objective is to protect a vulnerable adult. 'Preventative work' is another term which is not given enough attention and certainly the whole concept of prevention is not addressed nearly enough. This is due to the fact that with stretched resources most organisations are responding to crises, and crisis intervention work is the 'norm' rather than preventative work. The circular which accompanied the dissemination of *No Secrets* did mention prevention:

> All agencies will need to collaborate closely on developing their local codes of practice so that they can deal effectively with incidents of adult abuse. In doing so they should whenever possible endeavour to prevent abuse from occurring in the first place. (DOH (20th March 2000) Circular HSC 2000/007)

I would like the reader to be certain that in talking about adult abuse work I am implicitly talking about adult protection.

References

Department of Health (20th March 2000) Circular HSC 2000/007

Department of Health (2000) *No Secrets: Guidance on developing and implementing multi-agency policies and procedures to protect vulnerable adults from abuse.* London: HMSO.

Pritchard, J. (1995) *The Abuse of Older People.* 2nd Edition London: Jessica Kingsley Publishers.

Pritchard, J. (1996) *Working with Elder Abuse: A Training Manual for Home Care, Residential and Day Care Staff.* London: Jessica Kingsley Publishers.

Chapter 1

Developing Training Within Organisations

In the Introduction to this guide, I explained that there seems to be a move towards developing pools of trainers in order to ensure that large numbers of staff within or across organisations can be trained on adult abuse. These pools tend to concentrate on providing basic awareness training. In this chapter I want to focus on how training on adult abuse should be developed as an ongoing programme. In my working life I do get a view of what is happening around the UK and there are great differences between organisations. I would also like to share my own personal viewpoints which have developed over the years as a result of providing training myself to all sorts of staff groups but also from my role as consultant in developing training programmes.

Objectives of the Organisation

A fundamental question for anyone given the task of organising training is:

- 'What are the aims and objectives of the organisation in providing this training?'

This may seem to be a simplistic and perhaps obvious question, but I do not believe enough time and thought goes into considering it. Is the organisation putting on training because it *has* to do so or is it really committed to developing workers to their full potential? These questions lead onto other questions:

- 'Does the organisation want to provide basic training so that workers become equipped to do the job?'

and/or

- 'Do they want workers to become reflective practitioners?'

What I am leading to is the final question:

- 'Are there any hidden agendas?'

If an adult abuse trainer is already working within the organisation, then s/he is likely to have some understanding of the culture and politics that exist. However, if it is an outside trainer who is coming in, this knowledge is often lacking and can result in training being affected by the fact that participants start to offload their dissatisfaction onto the trainer. It is very important for the trainer to ensure this does not get out of hand and take over the session.

Before developing a training programme, the organisation itself needs to consider a number of issues, which are summarised in the checklist on the next page and could be used as an agenda for any development meeting. Some of the issues will need further planning and work before the answers are clear.

Organising training

At the current time, many organisations have to develop their own individual training programmes. Decisions have to be made by the organisation concerned about the training programme, that is, the courses that will be offered on adult abuse and their duration. In the current economic climate, many organisations are faced with budget constraints and, as adult abuse is not statutory work, very often it is not given the priority it deserves. Workers often feel frustrated that they only get the odd day's training here and there on adult abuse. In contrast, child protection workers are usually systematically trained and rolling training programmes are well planned with regular courses lasting anything from two days through to a full working week.

It is important for someone within the organisation to be given a lead role to develop a training programme for adult abuse and to work out exactly how many workers need the training, but also to identify their individual training needs, i.e. undertake a proper training needs analysis. I see around the UK that the strategies being developed for providing training in this subject area do vary tremendously.

Checklist of questions organisations need to ask themselves

- Why is adult abuse training needed in this organisation?

- Who needs to be trained?

- How many staff are we talking about?

- Will this training be done in-house only or in an inter-agency way?

- Who will take the lead for developing training/a training strategy?

- Who will do the training, i.e. staff within the organisation or an outside trainer?

- Shall we develop a pool of trainers?

- If training is to be done within the organisation, will staff be trained:

    (i)   within/across staff groups

    (ii)   across service user groups/specialisms

    (iii) with managers and workers together?

- Which individual courses should be provided?

- What are the course objectives and the learning outcomes?
  (This needs to be stated clearly for all participants but particularly for those who are undertaking National Vocational Qualifications.)

- How many courses will there be?

- How many participants should be included in each course?

- What will the costs be?

- Is there a budget limit?

- How will the training programme/courses/trainers be evaluated?

- Who will evaluate the training programme/courses/trainers?

- How often will the training programme be reviewed?

Organisations must acknowledge that workers are going to have different levels of knowledge and expertise, and consequently their training needs will vary. Managers have a responsibility to identify their workers' development and training needs; this is a fundamental function of the supervision process. Efficient systems need to be set up so that these needs can be fed back to the organisation's training section. In some organisations, workers have individual training profiles which can be used to identify training needs, evaluate courses, monitor development and systematically keep a record of courses undertaken.

Some organisations will internally prioritise staff who need the training. For example, within a social services department social workers who are going to be involved in investigations might be given priority over a home care assistant. I have never agreed with this as I think many groups of staff (like home care, residential/day care staff) are given low priority because they are not seen to be as important as the 'qualified staff'. I have said for a long time that it is these groups of staff who are more likely to pick up signs of abuse and also to receive a disclosure (Pritchard 1996). This is because they spend so much time with service users and can build up knowledge and trust. Consequently, they should be given appropriate training to alert them to the fact that they could have a very important role to play in identification of abuse, and courses must be developed in order to provide them with the knowledge and tools needed to carry out this role.

Similarly within the health services, I have always been concerned that certain groups of medical staff do not received specialised training on adult abuse, e.g. nurses and doctors in Accident and Emergency departments. It is my belief that many abuse cases are missed because staff are not aware of adult abuse, unlike staff who work in children's hospitals and have undertaken specialised training in child protection work.

It is possible to learn from the child protection field where training is undertaken in a multi-disciplinary way. This has to happen in the adult abuse field too, but until sufficient funding is put into promoting such training, it is unlikely to happen on a large scale. Where organisations have attempted to provide training in this way, there are often problems in organising and funding the training programme, because so many workers need to be trained. Special development posts have been created in some organisations to co-ordinate such training, but such progress is not as yet widespread. Again I do not believe this will happen on a large scale until adult abuse work is given the recognition it deserves. When the guidance *No Secrets* was launched in

March 2000, the Government stated under Section 7 of the Local Authority Social Services Act that:

> The aim of 'No Secrets' is to ensure that key local agencies, particularly but not solely health, social services and the police, are able to work together to protect vulnerable adults from abuse by developing local multi-agency policies and procedures…The co-ordinating role falls to social services departments… Directors of Social Services will be expected to ensure that the local multi-agency codes of practices are developed and implemented by 31st October 2001.
>
> (DOH Circular HSC 2000/007)

It is not enough to develop codes of practice alone; organisations must develop appropriate training programmes.

In the meantime, training will be developed according to how training sections within organisations are currently organised. Larger organisations may have training sections that are divided into specialisms related to service-users (e.g. children and families, mental health, adults with physical/sensory disability, adults with learning disabilities, older people) or to staff groups (e.g. home care, residential sector) or subjects (e.g. community care, National Vocational Qualification [NVQ]). Consequently, adult abuse may be incorporated into other training courses, but often this means only a very short session (maybe one or two hours) is devoted to the subject. Hence, my argument for one person to be given the lead to develop a training programme solely for adult abuse work.

In order to promote inter-agency working, the lead people within each organisation need to communicate. In some areas this is currently being done through local adult protection committees or working groups that have been formed solely to promote inter-agency training. As a result of *No Secrets* it may be that more agencies meet through the recommended multi-agency management committees. (p15, DOH 2000).

The dilemmas facing organisers of training

I have written elsewhere (Pritchard 1999) about the dilemmas facing training officers when organising training on adult abuse and some of the dilemmas may have been resolved by the organisation if it has prepared well (see checklist on page 20). A training officer (or lead person) has many issues to consider but the initial ones will be:

- who to train and who should be trained first/given priority
- identification of trainers
- course content
- duration of courses
- numbers of courses
- costs/budget.

To summarise, it is necessary to decide whether to train workers (both purchasers and providers):

- within specialisms (e.g. all staff working with: (i) adults with learning disability; (ii) adults with physical/sensory disability; (ii) adults with mental health problems; (iii) older people)
- within staff groups (e.g. social workers; home care; residential staff)
- managers and workers together
- across agencies.

There are pros and cons for each one of these. Workers sometimes feel 'safer' if they train with people they know – within their own staff group or within their own specialism. Recently, a residential worker said to me that when training alongside social workers she felt like 'a fish out of water'. The negative side, if one plays it safe, is that there is not then a sharing of knowledge across specialisms. I believe it is helpful to have some understanding about other service user groups. Dangerous practices can develop if a worker becomes so entrenched in working with only one service user group; it is necessary to widen one's knowledge base or else things can be missed. This is my argument for workers in children and families teams undertaking adult abuse training and workers in the adult sector undertaking child protection training. In some cases, there can be two social workers visiting a family because there are children at risk in the household, but there may also be other adults in need or at risk as well. Workers need to broaden their focus.

I personally find it good to train managers and workers together. If one separates grass-roots workers and managers, then the trainer starts hearing two sides to the story; there is often criticism on both sides. For example, workers will say that they are not getting the time they need to do investigations properly. Managers will say that workers are not coming to them for advice. I find on most courses many questions are asked about the interpretation of the local policy and procedures, e.g.

When does work become a formal adult abuse investigation?; What is the difference between a strategy meeting and a case conference?; When should the police be contacted? It is helpful to have managers and workers together to discuss these issues. Managers sometimes do not give training the priority it deserves because of other work pressures. I think it is crucial that *all* managers should undertake the same training as their workers on adult abuse, so that they know how they are being trained and there can be consistency in practice.

Ideally, I think we should be promoting inter-agency training. What is daunting is the number of workers who need to be trained within a local area. Within large cities this is an absolute nightmare and hence the reason for developing pools of trainers. One of the most positive things to come out of inter-agency training is the way in which different workers start communicating and foundations are laid for future liaison.

When we talk about inter-agency training people always think of the 'usuals', e.g. social services, health, police. It is necessary to think more broadly; that is, not just of personnel from the statutory sector. I have found that housing departments or local housing associations are often forgotten. In an ideal world, organisers of training should include workers from voluntary agencies and the independent sector (and we should not just be thinking of residential homes here; for example, there are many private home care agencies now).

I also have concerns that certain staff within health are not always considered for training on adult abuse. Again, it is important that the hierarchy engage in training; no one should be afraid to admit that they have little knowledge in this area of work. Psychologists and psychiatrists are often needed for assessment purposes, e.g. to give information about self-harming behaviours, attempted suicide and mental capacity. A recent research project found that many workers did not have knowledge about the long-term effects of abuse, e.g. eating disorders (Pritchard 2000). Staff who are often not automatically included in adult abuse training are dieticians. Victims often disclose when they are doing something intimate; therefore, physiotherapists, speech therapists etc are people who should receive training.

Another common problem concerns general practitioners (GPs); how do you get them to come on adult abuse training? I have not got any brilliant solutions to this problem. Again, the difficulty is that adult abuse work is not seen as a priority for many GPs. This is worrying, as GPs and their practice nurses could be crucial in iden-tifying cases of adult abuse, but they also could have a role to play in monitoring cases. More effort needs to be put into working with and encouraging GPs to participate in training sessions that may be offered to them.

The adult abuse training programme

It is not enough just to provide basic raising-awareness courses when a policy has been developed. Good practice would indicate that an ongoing training programme for adult abuse should be developed. As I have explained earlier, it is not my intention to discuss the development of advanced courses in this guide as I believe that this needs to be undertaken by experienced trainers. In Chapter 5 I shall be discussing in depth the content of a basic raising awareness course, but it might be useful to state here what I think an overall training programme on adult abuse should include. Table 1.1 makes some suggestions regarding the types of courses which could be part of such a plan.

All staff who work with vulnerable adults should have a basic raising-awareness course followed later by an investigation course, then intervention course (that is, how to undertake long-term work with victims and abusers). It is important that all staff groups realise that they could have a supportive role to play in the investigation process or an active role in a protection plan because they are working with a victim or abuser. Some staff believe they will never be involved in an adult abuse investigation; therefore, they do not see the need for training. It needs to be explained to these workers that they could have a supportive role to play. For example, a victim may disclose to a care worker in a voluntary-supported accommodation project and then want that particular worker present when they are interviewed by a social worker and the police.

Briefing sessions

In some organisations I have been asked to present briefing sessions when a new policy has been developed or a policy has been re-written. This is often seen as part of training, but I would not define it as 'proper training'. I think briefing sessions can be extremely useful if they are presented in a creative way, but workers attending such sessions need to be clear that it is *not* a formal training session. The aim of a briefing session is to familiarise workers with a new policy/procedure.

Table 1.1 Adult Abuse Courses

Type of course	Subject areas to include
1. Basic raising-awareness	Definitions of adult abuse. Signs and symptoms. Procedures.
2. Investigation	More in-depth training on procedures. Process of investigation. Techniques/methods (to include interviewing).
3. Intervention	Long-term work with victims and abusers.
4. Legislation	Legislation that can be used in adult abuse work. Criminal and civil actions.
5. Handling disclosure	How to receive disclosure without corrupting the evidence.
6. Recording and developing protection plans.	Back to basics regarding good recording technique. How to develop and write proper protection plans.
7. Chairing and/or participating in case conferences	Purpose of case conferences. Preparation. How to present information/behave. Format/agenda. Dealing with difficult situations. Analysing group dynamics.
8. Case review days	Updating on local and national developments. Review of cases and practice.

© Jacki Pritchard 2001

Information sheets

I discuss in Chapter 4 the importance of disseminating information about courses *before* they take place. On pages 27 and 28 I give some examples of typical course information sheets.

ADULT ABUSE: RAISING-AWARENESS COURSE

Date:

Time:

Venue:

Trainer:

Objectives

The aim of the course is to raise awareness about adult abuse; that is, to be clear that abuse of a vulnerable adult is an important issue which needs to be confronted by *all* professionals. This course will help participants to:

- consider what constitutes abuse (both in the community and institutional settings)
- develop skills in recognising abuse
- know what to do when abuse is suspected/identified.

Participation

There have been many developments in working with adult abuse since 1991. Participants will be informed about national developments and practices (in particular, policies and guidelines which exist within the UK); recent work and proposals regarding identifying abuse; and the law. Throughout the course attention will be given to the issues of confidentiality and professional boundaries.

Please note: this is a very practical course so participants will be expected to engage in group discussion and practical exercises (to be carried out in pairs and small groups).

Learning outcomes

By the end of the course participants will have:

- raised their awareness on the whole issue of adult abuse
- developed skills to be able to recognise signs and symptoms of adult abuse
- examined values and attitudes in regard to working with adult abuse
- an overview of legislation available
- a good working knowledge of what constitutes good practice
- a clear understanding of the local policy and procedure.

Figure 1.1

ADULT ABUSE: INVESTIGATION COURSE

Date:

Time:

Venue:

Trainer:

Objectives

To enable participants to further develop their skills in working with adult abuse. Course participants should be attending the investigation course in order to develop skills in carrying out investigations into adult abuse, but also to consider long-term work with victims and abusers.

Participation

A variety of methods will be used to help participants to develop their skills further in this area of work.

Please note: this is a very practical-based course so participants will be expected to engage in group discussion, practical exercises (to be carried out in pairs and small groups) and role play.

Learning outcomes

By the end of the course participants will have:

- raised their awareness further on the whole issue of adult abuse

- developed skills in identifying injuries

- a clear understanding about working in a multidisciplinary way

- a clear understanding about their own role in working with abuse

- thought about sexual abuse in depth and gathering evidence

- a clear understanding of the procedures involved in carrying out an investigation

- developed appropriate interviewing skills

- given more thought to what constitutes good practice in investigations

- gained knowledge about monitoring tools and developing protection plans

- developed confidence in working with abuse, both in the short term and long term.

Figure 1.2

© Jacki Pritchard 2001

Length of courses

I believe very strongly that any course on adult abuse should not be too long in duration, purely because it is a very emotive subject. If someone has never considered the topic before it can be emotionally draining and s/he may switch off. It is important not to bombard course participants with too much information. I constantly have to remind myself about this fact, when I feel frustrated by time constraints and I want to give people as much information as possible in the time allocated to me.

Ideally I think training programmes should be organised into modules over a specific period of time. I have experience of delivering short courses over a 4–6 week period, where participants come back once a week or it can be spread out over a longer period, perhaps six months, where participants come back once a month. The latter is more helpful in giving participants time to reflect on practice and bring back issues for discussion.

People can obtain information on a module, go back to work to put the theory into practice, then return to the following module with the objective of feeding back on practice and learning another element. I prefer this way of training rather than having courses which last two, three or four days together; the aftermath of which is that the participants and the trainer are absolutely exhausted. There is only so much information a person can digest and reflect on in a set period of time. Table 1.2 gives some suggestions about duration of courses and is followed by some of my tips for trainers.

Table 1.2 Duration of Courses

Course	Duration
Briefing sessions – when a new policy/ procedure is launched or relaunched	Half day
Basic raising-awareness	Half or full day
Investigation	1–2 days
Intervention (Long-term work)	1–2 days
Legislation	Half day
Handling disclosure	Half day
Recording/developing protection plans	Half day
Case conferences	Full day
Case review days	Full day

TRAINER TIPS

- **Full-day courses** should run 9.30 a.m. to 4.00 p.m at the latest. People are just too tired to carry on if the course goes on late.

- **Half-day courses** are an ideal duration if they run 9.30 a.m to 1.00 p.m. Mornings are always better because workers often get caught up in other things and then do not turn up for afternoon sessions.

- **Breaks** should be organised and of a duration that allows people to get their drinks and have a chance to unwind; they should not be rushed.

- **Lunch breaks** should be short rather than long. People often like to negotiate with the trainer for shorter lunch breaks and earlier finish time. This is preferable to sitting around dragging out the lunch-hour (especially if there is nowhere to go locally). Obviously if participants have to go out to get their food, a full hour may be needed. If this is not the case, then training organisers need to think about time-tabling in a shorter lunch break.

In Chapters 4 and 5 attention will be given to preparation for training and developing the content of a basic awareness course on adult abuse. Organisations also have a responsibility to evaluate the training which is being provided and this will be discussed in full in Chapter 8.

References

Department of Health (2000) *No Secrets: Guidance on Developing and Implementing Multi-Agency Policies and Procedures to Protect Vulnerable Adults from Abuse.* London: HMSO.

Department of Health (20th March 2000) Circular HSC 2000/007.

Pritchard, J. (1999) 'Lessons learnt in working with elder abuse in the last decade' in Pritchard, J. (ed) *Elder Abuse Work: Best Practice in Britain and Canada.* London: Jessica Kingsley Publishers.

Pritchard, J. (1996) *Working with Elder Abuse: A Training Manual for Home Care, Residential and Day Care Staff.* London: Jessica Kingsley Publishers.

Pritchard, J. (2000) *The Needs of Older Women: Services for Victims of Elder Abuse and Other Abuse.* Bristol: Policy Press.

Chapter 2

Selecting a Pool of Trainers

In the organisations where I have trained pools of trainers, the selection of trainers has not been very systematic; it has generally been on an ad hoc basis, i.e. whoever volunteers ends up doing the job. I am not saying this happens everywhere, but I want to discuss in this chapter what *should* happen. There needs to be a process by which a pool can be recruited, developed and maintained effectively.

Developing pools of trainers is a fairly new development in the adult abuse field and often there is an expectation that not enough people will volunteer to become trainers. The selection of trainers for a pool should be undertaken through a proper process; that is, there should be a thorough recruitment process. Being a trainer is a job which carries many responsibilities with it and when training on adult abuse there are complex pressures and difficulties (which will be discussed in the following chapters). It is crucial that the right people are selected, otherwise the training provided might not be good, effective or worthwhile. Also, if a trainer does not have the necessary skills, participants could be damaged in the process of training on adult abuse.

It is important to dismiss some myths I hear frequently about being a trainer and providing courses:

- 'Being a trainer is an easy life because you just keep saying and doing the same thing.'

- 'Anyone can be a trainer.'

Being a trainer is in fact extremely hard because it is physically, mentally and emotionally draining. I also think it is a vocation in life and not everybody has the skills or personality to do it. It worries me when I see people who are tired of their job (typical scenario is a burnt-out social worker or nurse) and they think that becoming a trainer will be an escape route (either by moving into a vacancy in the training section or going independent). You should become a trainer because you want to train people in order to develop them and sow the seeds for good practice. You can become a trainer when you know that you have the knowledge, required skills, commitment and enthusiasm; that is, you should have the real desire to train – it should not be an alternative to doing something else.

I know many people will disagree with me, but I do not believe that 'if you are a natural trainer, you can train on anything'. I know that some training sections within organisations move personnel around to deliver courses on subjects, which they know little about. The fundamental expectation is that you 'learn' the subject. To be an effective trainer I believe you have to feel passionately about the subject as well as knowing it back to front. If the trainer is uninterested in the subject or bored by it, then the delivery of courses is unlikely to be stimulating.

A person who is interested in becoming a full-time trainer needs to have some practice runs at it before they commit to it fully. Some managers and practitioners within organisations have a responsibility for training their staff, so may get the opportunity to actually train within their current job. Practitioners may have a special interest or expertise in a particular subject and be asked to give short presentations to groups; all of which are good learning and testing-out experiences. However, before fully committing to training, I think people do need to run full-day courses to see if they can hack it. Short sessions never give you the true taste of experiencing life as a trainer. Also, training on the odd day is nothing like training for five days a week, which I do not think anyone should do anyway. I think if you train more than three days each week, you are not going to give people your best. You are just too tired.

I have always said that training is like acting – you are performing in front of an audience. The actor has to be entertaining; similarly the trainer has to be able to present the plot clearly and communicate in a way which engages the participants. Some people just have not got the personality to do this. Exercise 2.1 may help potential trainers to think about whether they have the necessary qualities to make a good trainer.

WHAT MAKES A GOOD TRAINER?

Objective

To help people who are thinking about becoming a trainer analyse what qualities are needed to be an effective trainer.

Participants

This exercise is to be undertaken by individuals, but a mentor is also needed.

Equipment

Paper and pen.

Task

Stage 1

The individual should think about training courses they have attended in the past, but in particular think about the trainers, both good and bad. Make a list of the good ones first of all and list *why* they were good, i.e. what it was about them that made them effective. Make a second list for bad trainers and focus on why they were not good.

Stage 2

Make a list of qualities you have which you think would make you a good trainer. Make a second list about the doubts you have about yourself.

Stage 3

Discuss all the lists with the mentor, that is, someone who has experience in training.

Stage 4

Make the decision: are you going to try to become a trainer?

Table 2.1 lists some typical comments written by course participants on evaluation forms about a range of trainers in different organisations. It may be helpful to think about some of these when doing Exercise 2.1.

Table 2.1 Good and bad trainers

What was good	*What was bad*
Lively personality	Too domineering
Charismatic	Talked too much
Able to listen	Full of themselves
Caring	Used posh words
Knows the subject	Boring
Has real experience	Talks in a flat tone
Approachable	Never smiled
I could talk to him	Too serious
I didn't feel embarrassed asking questions	Detached from the real world
She didn't make me feel stupid	Not done the job for years
She understood how I felt	Didn't give us enough time; rushed us
Clear – spoke in English not jargon	Talked down to us
Explained what he meant	She was hard going
Encouraged us	Didn't understand the words he used
Could have a joke alongside the serious stuff	

As well as being a performer on view, there are so many other things that can make the trainer tired. For example, you have to constantly:

- be alert to what is happening within the group

- answer and field questions

- deal with difficult participants

- make sure you get all the material in, so you have achieved the objectives and learning outcomes by the end of the course

- react – a trainer never knows what is going to be thrown at them; s/he has to be able to think quickly on his/her feet and react to situations that present themselves.

Everyone wants to meet the ideal trainer and have them in the pool, but how do you go about it?

Developing a pool of trainers

If an organisation decides that it needs a pool of trainers to train a large number of staff, further basic questions need to be asked before going ahead (see page 36 overleaf).

Developing a pool of trainers: Some basic questions for organisations

- How many trainers are needed in the pool?

- What is the maximum/minimum number? (Organisations have to be realistic about how many trainers can be recruited, trained, supported and by whom.)

- How many should we recruit initially?

- Will recruitment be ongoing?

- What happens if people drop out? (which they often do!)

- How do we replace them?

- How will they be recruited?

- Who is going to train them?

- Who is going to support them?

- Who is going to monitor and evaluate their performance?

- What happens if a trainer is not performing satisfactorily?

- Do we need time-limited contracts?

© Jacki Pritchard 2001

The selection process

After the initial planning stages, there needs to be a very clear selection process and stages need to be followed:

SELECTION PROCESS

- Deciding criteria for selection – equivalent to developing a job description and personal specification.

- Advertisement – be clear about what is expected of the trainer re time commitment, training for the pool, provision of courses, support, evaluation of performance.

- Meetings – it is helpful to convene meetings so that potential trainers can be given specific information about the pool and how it will be developed.

- Formal interview – to include a presentation on some aspect of adult abuse.

Whoever is responsible for developing a pool of trainers needs to start the selection process by asking:

- 'What are we looking for in a trainer on adult abuse?'

Competencies have gained a high profile in recent years and the selection process begins by thinking about what competencies are required of a trainer. From this a personal specification and a job description could be developed. This may seem very formal, especially when the trainers in a pool will probably be doing this in addition to their day-to-day job. Nevertheless, it is important to have some degree of formality so that the 'job' is taken seriously; it is not viewed as 'just another add-on'; 'something different to do to break the monotony'; 'it'll be good for the CV'. It concerns me that very often the process is to ask for volunteers who are interested in forming a pool to attend informal meetings and then a training-the-trainers course.

There is lot of debate about competencies and the value of competence-based training (Ashworth and Saxton 1990; Hyland 1995; Yelloly and Henkel 1995); certainly thought needs to be given to the competencies required by a trainer but in addition specific requirements need to be developed concerning:

- values

- knowledge

- skills

- training.

Below I list questions regarding what I would like to know about a person who was interested in training on adult abuse:

FINDING OUT ABOUT A POTENTIAL TRAINER

- What is his/her attitude to abuse in general?

- How does s/he define abuse?

- Has s/he a personal history of abuse? If s/he has, will this affect his/her delivery of training?

- Has s/he direct experience of working with abuse?

- Have s/he experience of handling disclosure?

- What is his/her level of emotional maturity?

- Has s/he had any training on abuse; if so to what level?

- Of which service-user groups does s/he have experience?

- Does s/he have any previous experience of training?

Finding out as much information as possible about the potential trainer's values and attitudes towards abuse is of paramount importance. This must be drawn out in interview, as must a personal history of abuse that might affect the running of courses. If issues have not be resolved for the trainer personally, all sorts of triggers, memories and difficulties could arise when discussions or disclosures take place on a course. I am *not* saying victims of abuse should not train; I am suggesting that there needs to be clarification about whether the victim has healed and has the ability to help and train others to understand about abuse and why it happens. They should not be bringing their own agendas to the course. There are many organisations that provide training on domestic violence and abuse using input from victims them-

INTERVIEW SUBJECT AREAS

Values

- Value base – socially constructed, holistic, client-centred?
- Anti-discriminatory practice
- Anti-oppressive practice
- Equal opportunities
- Rights
- Responsibilities
- Collaboration
- Sharing of power; power relationships
- Openness; honesty; confidentiality
- User focus
- User needs
- User involvement

Knowledge

- Human development
- Child abuse
- Domestic violence
- Adult abuse
- Definitions of adult abuse
- Recognising abuse – signs and symptoms
- Effects of abuse – short- and long-term
- Behaviours, e.g. challenging, self-harm, suicidal
- Theories – abuse and violence – why does it happen?
- Interventions
- Local policies/procedures
- Legal matters
- Legislation
- Multi-disciplinary working – what does it mean; how do you achieve it?

Skills

- Presentation
- Listening
- Responding
- Communication
- Behavioural
- Interpersonal
- Reflective
- Analytical
- Observational
- Writing/recording
- Managing emotions
- Managing boundaries, e.g. own experiences, other people's, disclosure, confidentiality
- Managing anger, aggression, upset
- Relating personal and work experience
- Transfer of skills
- Dealing with acceptance/ tolerance/resistance

Training

- How adults learn
- Methods of teaching
- Group learning/group dynamics
- Requirements (e.g. CCETSW, NVQ)

selves. Many victims become successful trainers. However, if they have not dealt with certain issues themselves, there is the danger that they may use the training forum for their own purposes. I am advocating caution by striving for thorough assessment in interview.

In developing a personal specification, an organisation can use Exercise 2.2 on the facing page to think about what they require in a trainer.

The interview

Having decided what it wants in a trainer, the organisation then has to decide how it is going to find out if a worker has the specified requirements. This is the hard part. Interviews are very false situations because some people can excel at interview and others are really bad at presenting themselves (perhaps because of nerves). A decision must be made regarding the format of interviews. Giving a presentation is crucial when considering someone for a training job.

On page 41 I have listed some typical subject areas which need to be addressed in interview; these have been identified by organisations when undertaking Exercise 2.2 (using their own terminology). This list can be used for discussion when deciding how to conduct the interview.

Post interview

After a person has been selected, s/he has to be trained, supported and evaluated. This will be the subject matter for the following chapters. It needs to be emphasised that some people find that they are just not cut out to be trainers. This should not be seen as a failure. None of us can be good at everything; we have to find out what we are good at and follow that path.

References

Ashworth, P. and Saxton, J. (1990) 'On 'competence', *Journal of Further and Higher Education 14*, 2, 8–25

Hyland, T. (1995) 'Behaviourism and the meaning of competence' in P. Hodkinson and M. Issitt (eds) *The Challenge of Competence*. London: Cassell.

Yelloly, M. and Henkel, M. (1995) *Learning and Teaching in Social Work: Towards Reflective Practice*. London: Jessica Kingsley Publishers.

WHAT ARE WE LOOKING FOR IN A TRAINER?

Objective

To help organisations think about qualities and requirements that are needed in a trainer and to develop a personal specification.

Participants

This exercise will be undertaken by the group of people who are responsible for developing a pool of trainers. If the group is large (i.e. more than six), it may be preferable to break into smaller groups and then feed back before developing a personal specification.

Equipment

Flipchart paper and pens

Time

1–2 hours

Task

The groups are asked to discuss and then list the requirements under the following four headings:

    (1)   values

    (2)   skills

    (3)   knowledge

    (4)   training.

A personal specification will then be written.

Chapter 3

Training and Supporting the Trainers

Organisations that are going to develop a pool of trainers to provide basic awareness training on adult abuse must take time to consider how they are going to recruit suitable practitioners and managers to the pool. In the previous chapter we gave consideration to *who* should train, but that does not solve completely the problem of obtaining the right people for the pool. When I have been involved in training pools, it has become clear very early on in the process that people have not really had much information about what is expected of them and crucially the time commitment. It is important to be clear at the outset, otherwise potential trainers will fall by the wayside.

Releasing staff and contracts

Most workers, whichever discipline they work in, are already over-stretched and under a great deal of pressure to do their day-to-day jobs. Therefore, when an organisation asks for nominations from workers to become trainers the response is often poor. Workers may have the inclination to volunteer, but do not do so because of the current pressures inflicted upon them. Depending on the amount of training to be provided by each individual, organisations need to explore the possibility of reducing workloads; people should not be expected to do it on top of everything else (which is the normal expectation). Another harsh reality is that some managers may not even inform workers about the possibility of becoming a trainer, because they know it will affect other members of the team, workloads, rotas etc. Therefore, the opportunity is never made public. Another side of the situation is that an organisation says that there *must* be so many trainers nominated and people are then forced into the position. This is not satisfactory as these particular trainers may not be committed to doing the job and see it as a burden.

Whatever the situation, contracts should be made with workers who are going to be part of a pool. Copies of the contract should be made available to the worker's line manager, so everyone is clear about the commitment to be undertaken. Contracts should cover:

- release from work

- number and duration of training days for training the worker to be in the pool

- number of days training to be provided by the worker once they have been trained for the pool

- number of days for formally reflecting on and evaluating the worker's performance.

Information

At the outset, organisations must be up-front and honest about what will be involved if someone commits to becoming a trainer; it is important that both managers and workers receive this information. Information which is initially circulated needs to address the following questions:

- How will the pool be formed? Will it be informal (i.e. whoever volunteers after an initial meeting) or formal (i.e. by interview to fit specific criteria)?

- How many days will be provided to train the trainers and over what period of time?

- How many training courses will the trainer be expected to provide over a year?

- Will there be ongoing support/training for the trainer?

All this information should be provided in written form in the first instance but meetings also need to be organised in an attempt to attract staff. Whoever leads these sessions needs to be clear and specific. Workers will not sign up if everything is too vague and they are told 'We haven't quite decided about that yet' or 'We'll take that back for further discussion'. Workers need to know that it *is* a huge commitment; a lot of time and effort are needed if they have never provided any training before. The reality is that many potential trainers do a lot of the preparation and learning, which is needed to become a trainer, in their own time rather than in work time. It can be a steep learning curve.

Training the trainers

Many organisations develop training-the-trainers sessions in order to 'teach' the trainers about what they have to provide on training courses. It is important not to rush in and just give the course content to the trainers; some preparatory work needs to be undertaken. The workers in the pool will be coming from a variety of backgrounds; they will also have different levels of experience, skills and confidence. There needs to be some equivalent to 'team-building' so that members of the pool will be able to voice their fears and anxieties during the training sessions. The leader needs to set aside time on the agenda for the group to get to know each other, but also for the leader to find out the level of knowledge and expertise held within the group. If time allows, the leader should also ascertain *how* the individuals learn best by using specific questionnaires and exercises (e.g. from Honey and Mumford 1982). However, in most organisations time is very limited and the leader may have been briefed to 'teach the course content' (for discussion about course content see Chapter 5). Nevertheless, the leader should aim to cover:

- experience and skills of trainers within the pool
- fears and anxieties
- course content
- learning the material
- handouts/other materials
- presentation styles and skills.
- rehearsal.

Building confidence

Many people come to a training-the-trainers course and are very nervous indeed. So it is important that the leader helps to make them feel relaxed and brings out the fact that they already have skills which can be utilised when in the trainer role. Exercise 3.1 can help with this in the early stages.

THE TREE EXERCISE

Objective

To help participants identify skills that they have and use in other work situations, which could help them in presenting training sessions.

Participants

Participants will work by themselves initially.

Time

10 minutes to work individually; 30 minutes to view the drawings and discuss.

Equipment

Paper, pens and blutak.

Task

On an A4 sheet of paper, participants are asked to draw a tree trunk with many branches stemming from it. They then have to add leaves to the branches. On each leaf they have to write a skill they possess that could be useful in a training session.

Feedback

After participants have completed their task, all the trees are put up on a wall. The leader will ask the group to comment on the skills they possess, then to identify skills which may be missing, but which are seen to be needed by a trainer.

Please note: participants should keep their trees safe as they may be used in future sessions and if they participate in Exercise 8.1. for evaluation purposes (see Chapter 8)

Deciding on the content of the course

Sometimes the content and format of the course will already have been decided before the trainers come together in the pool. This may have been decided by people 'higher up' or those given the lead to work on adult abuse (e.g. members of the local Adult Protection Committee, the Working Party who developed the current policy and procedure, or other key individuals such as training officers, independent consultants). In other circumstances, it may be left to the pool of trainers to decide how and what they are going to present. There may be a loose framework in terms of time and number of training days it is possible to fund in a given year. Where there is this freedom, the leader needs to add time to the programme to facilitate discussion on content and format and use of handouts. A word of caution is needed here. In my experience, the leader needs to be quite firm about the amount of time set to do this task. If there is no clear consensus between participants a lot of time can be wasted as the discussion goes round in circles. This discussion will be pursued further in Chapter 5.

Teaching the content of the course

There are numerous ways to train the trainers, and organisations need to explain the objectives and criteria, i.e. be clear what they want from the person being brought in to train and develop the pool. I believe there has to be some degree of flexibility, as the leader must adapt to the needs of the participants and the way they learn.

The leader must identify gaps in knowledge. It is not uncommon to find participants in a pool who have had no formal training on adult abuse themselves or have never worked on an abuse case. In these circumstances, these participants will need to be 'taught'. The two main areas where I have found knowledge to be lacking have been in regard to:

1. What constitutes abuse.

   Participants may have read the definitions in the local policy and procedure document, but may not be au fait with the detail under each category of abuse. Participants worry that they are not going to be clear enough themselves when they present information. There is often confusion regarding the overlap between categories. Therefore, it is crucial that participants become familiar with the definitions as stated in the local policy and procedure document.

2.   Recognising abuse

If the course requires the trainers to provide a session on signs and symptoms of abuse, similar problems arise. I have to say I have found this the most problematic area when training trainers. It is particularly difficult if a participant has little or no experience of working with abuse or s/he has little understanding of why abuse occurs. Hence my reason for believing that it is preferable for a trainer to have had some direct experience of working with abuse. No matter what level of experience a participant comes with, there has to be some degree of 'hard learning' in this area.

A potential trainer *must* realise that s/he is going to have to put in some personal time into learning material for the content of the course. S/he will have to be very familiar with the local policy and procedure document but also the leader should provide written materials and suggested reading lists without burdening the trainer with too much information (some suggested materials are given in the Appendix).

Working in pairs

Some pools decide that the trainers should be inter-changeable; that is, they should be able to co-train with anyone within the pool. This may be achievable once trainers become more experienced, but when they are inexperienced I believe it is better for two trainers to work together on a regular basis. As they become more familiar with the material they will also be getting to know each other – their weaknesses and strengths, reading the signs when one is uncomfortable, struggling, needs rescuing etc.

Once the pool of trainers have got to know each other, the leader may have a feel for who will work well together. Consideration needs to be given to achieving a good mix of experience, skills and presentation styles. The leader may discuss with the pool who they think would work well together and the potential audiences need to be considered. If basic awareness training is going to be undertaken on a multi-agency basis, then there should be a mix of trainers, e.g. social worker and nurse; police person and residential home manager. Other considerations may be in regard to character (extrovert and introvert) and gender mix.

Rehearsing

Rehearsals can be done in several ways depending on how comfortable or threatened the participants feel. Some participants may choose to rehearse outside of the formal training sessions. However, I feel it is very important for participants to 'practice' in front of each other and the leader. Some may feel very embarrassed and threatened, but at the end of the day they are going to have 'to go public'. To begin with I invite a participant to rehearse very small bits in short bursts – for example, introducing:

- him/herself

- the participants of the course

- the domestic arrangements, i.e. toilets, fire exits, break times etc

- the purpose of the course

- the programme

- the ground rules.

All the above can be done one at a time; participants taking it in turns. The participants who are observing are asked for constructive criticism and to pick up on any 'bad habits'. For example, we all have tendencies to use certain words too regularly or have certain body language which is distracting. It is important for each participant to get feedback on:

- clarity

- being loud enough or too quiet

- talking too quickly/too slowly

- body language.

When the pool has chosen who is going to work with whom, each pair need to meet and prepare for their sessions before rehearsing. The following decisions have to be made:

- Which teaching aids will be used (e.g. flipcharts, overhead projections, handouts, notes or cards for the trainer)?

- Who will present the different parts of the programme?

- Will this be inter-changeable over time so each trainer will be able to present each part of the course? (This is important if trainers are going to swop partners at a later date.)

Support

The pool of trainers needs to have ongoing support. The individual trainers need to have a contact person so that s/he can discuss any difficulties which may arise during the training courses. For the first couple of courses each pair of trainers should be shadowed by an experienced trainer, whose role will be to give support and advice, and to evaluate performance.

There should be ongoing support for the pool of trainers. Again, the trainers need to be able to discuss any problem with a specifically named person, but also many pools find it helpful to meet regularly (preferably with a facilitator) as a support group for each other. It is also important to review training programmes on a regular basis and to discuss developments or changes which are necessary. New trainers to the pool also need to be made to feel welcome and valued by the more established trainers.

Debriefing

As an independent trainer I find it very necessary to debrief after training courses and have set up systems so that I am well supported. If trainers are working in pairs, they can help each other to debrief and it is important to set time aside to do this. It is imperative for a trainer to be able wind down from the course. Trainers are like actors in that they have just given a performance and it is very necessary to come down from the 'high'. Working in pairs is helpful, but if someone has to work on his/her own it is crucial that there is a person to whom the trainer can off-load; even if it is only to say that the course has gone well.

Obviously if there have been problems on the course it is important that a trainer does not go home worrying about issues which need to be followed up. Consequently, it is helpful for each trainer to have a contact person who *is* going to be available at the end of the course if necessary.

Some courses will only be half-day sessions. I know because of pressures of work some trainers will book into their diaries appointments which immediately follow the end of the training course. This means they are dashing from the course straight into another arena; probably without having lunch or a break. They must make space to wind down. Line managers must also respect this need. Trainers who have run a training course should not be expected to go on shift half-an-hour after the course has finished. Apart from the fact that the trainer needs to wind down, very often the trainer will not finish as the course finishes. Often course participants will stay behind to discuss issues (or maybe disclose about abuse) so the trainer must not feel under pressure to leave because s/he has another commitment to go to.

TRAINER TIP

Always leave yourself one full hour after a course to:

- deal with anyone or anything that arises after the course has finished

- reflect and wind down before moving on to start something else.

Evaluation

Evaluation is considered in depth in Chapter 8, but mention of it must be made at this point too. Trainers within a pool do need to be evaluated on a regular basis and several methods of evaluation need to be undertaken. It is important for trainers to be observed and evaluated by someone independent, but written evaluations are also valuable. Within a course evaluation form, specific questions need to be asked about the trainer's:

- delivery of information

- presentation style

- teaching methods

- ability to answer questions

- ability to get people involved

- approachability

- use of materials.

After a long one-day course and certainly after a two-day course, a trainer can feel emotionally and physically drained. It is important to reflect on the day but s/he must develop ways of cutting off from the training day and each individual will have different ways of coping with this. I am aware that some trainers use the travelling time to get home as a winding down/cutting off period. They will use the time to reflect and then cut off. We all need different things to help us relax. I have to have complete silence in the car after a training course; I know colleagues who are the complete opposite – they have to have music blasting away. Some will go for a drink, others will go for a workout in the gym, others will sit and watch the soaps on TV! It is important to do a totally different activity.

Final comment

This chapter has shown the amount and depth of support which organisations must provide for trainers if they are to be valued and sustained. This is crucial not just for workers who are within the pool; the organisation must take responsibility for ensuring that outside trainers are also given appropriate support. As I have stated in earlier chapters, it is not enough for an organisation to develop a training programme on adult abuse and then do nothing else. So many different tasks have to be undertaken; a crucial one being the training and ongoing support for trainers working for the organisation. If trainers do not receive adequate support and validation, they will either give up or become burnt-out, very much in the same way as some workers do.

The framework for training the trainers

Training a pool of trainers should be a lengthy and ongoing process. If it is rushed, the trainers will not train effectively. Organisations need to take on board the framework on the next page (page 52) to develop an effective pool of trainers.

References

Honey, P. and Mumford, A. (1982) *The Manual of Learning Styles.* Maidenhead: Honey.

Framework and tasks

- Initial meeting:

   To give information about the pool of trainers and the future training programme.

- Selection process:

   Informal or formal.

- Training the trainers sessions:

   Organisations need to be clear about (i) number of sessions; (ii) duration; (iii) specific programme/agenda.

- Trainers to provide courses:

   Number to be decided and time-scale to be decided. Trainers to be shadowed for initial sessions.

- Each trainer needs a named contact person:

   The contact person will be available to support the trainer for debriefing or any difficulties which arise and need to be dealt with quickly.

- Feedback sessions after initial training courses:

   For trainers to feedback on how they have coped and to evaluate their training skills and the courses provided.

- Evaluation of trainers:

   Process to be decided by organisation.

- Rolling recruitment to pool:

   Organisations should decide whether they will continue to recruit to the pool and how they will actually do this in the future.

Chapter 4

Preparation

A great deal of thought needs to be given to practical matters before a training course takes place. This chapter will focus on some of the main issues that need to be addressed. For someone new to training, some of these things may never enter their head until it is too late. It is my hope that I will save new trainers some time, and help them to avoid some disastrous situations. All of these issues are pertinent to an individual trainer as well as to pools of trainers.

Venue

Some organisations may already have designated training rooms within their own office buildings or they may regularly use particular venues for a variety of reasons (e.g. low hire cost). When training on such a sensitive issue as adult abuse, it is crucial that the venue and the training environment are comfortable and meet a variety of needs.

The venue itself needs to be easily accessible. One should not assume that everyone has the use of a car. There will be many staff who have to rely on public transport and their feet; home care staff are a prime example. Ideally the venue should be close to a main bus route. Ample parking space is also important. Participants often walk in late because they 'have been driving around trying to find somewhere to park'; this can be very disruptive for the other participants as well as the trainer.

Therefore, organisers of training should ensure that detailed information is given to participants prior to the course regarding:

- location of the venue

- how to get there – by road, bus, rail

- car parking (e.g. on street; availability of car parks and whether they are short or long stay; hourly fees).

Training rooms

Over the years I have trained in some ghastly training rooms that have been totally unsuitable both for me as a trainer and for the participants. It is important that participants feel comfortable when they are training. I think this is even more important when they are being trained on difficult and emotive issues, such as adult abuse. If participants feel uncomfortable then they will not concentrate. Consideration needs to be given to the following:

- Size of room

  A trainer will have decided in advance how many people will be participating in the course. The training room should be large enough to accommodate the number without participants feeling cramped together.

- Furniture

  Chairs should be comfortable, not too low (many people suffer with back problems) and not positioned too closely together.

- Decoration, light and temperature

  It is not good to train in a gloomy environment. The décor is important; participants need to feel comfortable and safe. A training room needs to have a good amount of natural light. However, if there are a number of big windows in the room, the trainer should also check that the room is not on a main pathway; pedestrians outside can distract the participants.

  The trainer needs to be able to regulate the temperature of the room, because participants will have varying body temperatures. I am a particularly nesh person and I cannot concentrate if I am cold. Other people cannot concentrate when they are too hot. The trainer needs to familiarise him/herself with the heating/air conditioning systems in advance of the course taking place. Also s/he needs to check out which windows open and how they open (for example, do you need a special key to open them?). When extreme weather conditions are prevalent the trainer must have access to extra heaters (in winter) and efficient fans (in summer).

- Privacy/quiet

    I have already mentioned that windows and pedestrians outside can distract participants, but the trainer also needs to check out that privacy and quiet can be ensured throughout the course. For example, rooms which face onto a busy main road, can be very noisy. I know that sometimes training takes place within environments where service users are present (day room on a hospital ward; lounge within a residential home). These venues should be avoided if it is likely that service users may wander in and out of the training room.

- Number of rooms

    Another decision to be made before the course takes place concerns the number of rooms needed. If group work is to take place it may be necessary to have access to smaller break-off rooms. These rooms need to be close by; valuable time is often wasted if participants have to walk a distance to and from these rooms.

    When training on adult abuse, some participants may become distressed – an issue that will be addressed below and in Chapter 6. Therefore, it is important to have a room available where a participant can go if they need to take a break from the course.

- Equipment

    In my early days as a trainer I learnt many painful lessons regarding lack of equipment. One should never assume that if an organisation hires out training rooms it means that all the necessary equipment will be available. A trainer needs to be cautious and check out what is included in the hire price. Every trainer has his/her own preference for particular equipment; there follows on page 56 a general checklist. In addition a trainer also needs to prepare his/her own equipment which is to be taken to the venue. On page 57 is a list of possible suggestions.

Refreshments

I know that many organisations are struggling with budget cuts and training sections are usually the first to be hit. However, I think it is very important to value staff and one way of doing this is to make sure they are well looked after on training courses by providing good refreshments.

Equipment checklist

- Flipchart stand and paper

  Some organisations may provide the stand but expect you to bring your own paper so do check in advance.

- Flipchart pens

  It is always better to carry your own supply of flipchart pens, because often the pens available have run out or are drying up. When doing group work, participants often like to work with a variety of colours.

- White board and pens

  Again check the correct pens are available and take your own for the same reasons as stated above.

- Overhead projector and screen

  Check that the projector is working. A common fault is that bulbs have run out.

- Video/television

  It is always useful to check how these work *before* the course starts instead of fumbling about when you are ready to use the equipment.

Trainer's stuff

- Flipchart pens

    For reasons already stated above in Equipment checklist.

- Writing paper and pens

    Many participants may want to jot some notes down but often they have not come prepared to the course. So it is handy if the trainer has pens and paper readily available.

- Notebook for trainer

    The trainer may wish to make notes about people, incidents, what worked well/not very well. This can be done during break, lunchtime or at the end of the day.

- Blutak

- Sellotape and scissors

- Tissues

    There are occasions when participants become upset and some may need to have a good cry!

- Paracetomol/aspirin

    Time and time again I get asked for painkillers during courses; there may be all sorts of reasons for this. I have found that participants often do get headaches on abuse courses; they themselves say this is because they are concentrating so hard or finding it very emotional and stressful.

- Tampax

    Female trainers will get asked for these on frequent occasions.

Participants will feel welcomed if coffee and biscuits are available on arrival. It should also be remembered that some participants might not drink coffee or tea, so water or juice should be available as an alternative. I shall talk more below about flexibility and going at the group's pace, but I need to say here that I prefer to use venues where break times are not stipulated by the catering staff. My preference is to have drinks on tap so that I can stop and start to suit the needs of the participants. Lots of people (like myself) do not eat breakfast, so by mid morning they are starving and concentration levels can be affected. So biscuits should be provided with drinks at break times.

There is often a lot of resentment from the staff working in the adult sector if they see colleagues working in the children and families sector being provided with good lunches (which are paid for out of the Area Child Protection Committee budget) but they have to go out to buy their own lunches.

Length of the course

Every organisation will have its own ideas about how staff should be trained on adult abuse. Some training may be done in-house for different groups of staff, other courses will be run on a multi-agency basis. The dilemma for most organisations is having a vast number of staff who must be trained. It is crucial that *all* staff undertake some basic raising-awareness training. It has always been a major concern of mine that many front-line staff, who are usually the ones to hear a disclosure about abuse (namely workers from home care, day care, residential and supported accommodation settings) are not given priority on such courses. Another dilemma for organisations is the cost of such training. Consequently, it may be decided that basic raising-awareness training can be achieved in a half-day session. Organisations must be clear about what they are trying to achieve and not try to cram too much into a short session. Ideally, I think a raising-awareness session should be run over a full day.

The information sheet

Some organisations are very slack about the information they send out to course participants. This may be due to the training officer's lack of time or lack of administrative back-up. Nevertheless, a professional approach needs to be adopted. It has already been discussed above that detailed information is needed about the venue, but other information is also needed:

PRE-COURSE INFORMATION

- Date and time

  (Please note: make clear the difference between time for coffee on arrival and start time for course; participants get annoyed when they arrive for 9.00 a.m. only to find coffee and the course starts half an hour later.)

- Venue

- Trainer(s)

- Objectives of the course

- Learning outcomes

- Programme

- Statement about the subject matter

I would like to elaborate on the last point of the 'Pre-course Information list'. Sometimes I think it is important to make a statement in the pre-course information about the content of the course and that it may be a very emotive issue for some participants. I have trained people who have come on courses not knowing what they are going to be trained on; they have just been told by managers that they have to attend. This can be incredibly difficult for people who have been abused in the past or who are currently living in abusive situations. It is difficult to know how to warn people about the subject matter, because one does not want to raise anxieties unnecessarily.

People who work with abuse day in day out sometimes underestimate the effect on participants of hearing about abuse. I remember some years ago, training a group of home care staff on elder abuse. Whilst I was talking about defining sexual abuse, I noticed that one woman had literally turned white and I knew she was going to faint. She left the room and I went to see how I could help her. She told me that her father had sexually abused her when she was 10 years old and it was something I had said that had triggered off her memory. She said she had not thought about the abuse for the past 30 years. She had known she was coming on a course about 'elder abuse' but had never related this to sexual abuse. She had not made a connection. A trainer new to this area of work needs to be aware that all sorts of emotions and memories can be triggered in a training course on adult abuse. This is why it is important to set proper ground rules right at the beginning of the course.

Ground rules

Every trainer will have his/her own way of setting ground rules. I usually talk through mine on the flipchart:

Ground rule 1: space

As described above, some participants may find the course hard-going for any number of reasons. Abuse generally is a very emotive issue and if a participant has not really thought about the issue before then s/he can be upset by it. Although we do not have exact figures, we know that a large number of people in our society have been abused in childhood or in adulthood (and may well be continuing to live in such situations), so having to come on an adult abuse course can be extremely difficult for them. This ground rule allows any participant to be able to leave the room at any time to have some time and space to his/herself. This is the reason for having a spare room so that the participant knows that s/he has somewhere to go and will not be wandering around corridors or outside. It is important for the trainer to stress that the participant does not have to give an explanation to the trainer or the rest of the group why s/he wants some time out. It is also important to emphasise that the group agrees that no one will question the participant later on.

I have found that people do use this facility; they are not usually embarrassed at walking out because they have been given the permission to do so and know that other participants will not question them about it. I always check on the participant to see if they are OK, but I *never* ask them what is wrong; they know from Ground rule 2 that they can tell me if they wish to do so. If you are training alone then it is necessary to have some back-up facility – that is, a training officer to be around in case someone is very distressed and does not wish to be left alone. If there are two trainers it is easier, because one can check on the participant whilst the other continues with the course.

Ground rule 2: support

The trainer should offer support to all the participants. It should be made clear that if a participant wants to talk to the trainer during or after the course then this will be possible. I offer support both on work- and personal-related issues. I know some in-experienced trainers do not feel capable of offering this facility; therefore, the boundaries of support need to be stated clearly.

Ground rule 3: confidentiality

Most people understand that anything said within a training group is confidential. However, it is crucial that on any adult abuse training course there has to be a proviso. On such courses a trainer can pick up clues about abusive or bad practice, or s/he may actually be told about such practice. If this occurs, the trainer will have to break confidentiality. I shall use a simple example from my own experience.

Towards the end of a basic raising-awareness training course, a home care assistant said she wanted to disclose something to the group because she was feeling very upset. Having undergone the course she said she realised 'I am an abuser'. She had only been in the job a very short time and had been told by two district nurses that she must 'tie up' one of her older clients each night. The practice was that an older man was being tied to the cot sides of his bed with crepe bandages, which were put around his ankles and wrists. The home care assistant had believed this was all right because the nurses (whom she considered as 'professionals' and 'superior' to herself) had told her to do it. I spent time with this home care assistant after the course together with the training officer; she was extremely upset at what she had been doing but was also scared about the repercussions for herself ('for committing abuse') and the nurses, who she did not want to get into trouble. This home care assistant needed a great deal of support whilst an investigation took place.

Ground rule 4: respect

Again, another standard ground rule is about respecting other people's opinions. In abuse courses there is often a lot of debate and what comes to light are the differences in values and attitudes (especially when debating what constitutes abuse). Discussion often becomes loud and several people may interact at the same time. It is necessary for the trainer to emphasise the need for participants to listen, not to talk across each other, and to respect each person in the group.

Ground rule 5: keeping to time and having 'time outs'

The trainer needs to inform the group about timings (e.g. when to expect breaks – this is important for the smokers, who may get fidgety if they do not know when they can escape for their next cigarette!). If I am training over a full day I prefer to have two short breaks in the afternoon rather than one long one. People are always flagging after lunch (the infamous 'graveyard period'). I know some venues insist that breaks have to be at specific times but again I think it is important that a trainer goes at the group's pace.

I also have what I call 'time outs' or what several participants have renamed 'toilet stops'. Sometimes I am crucially aware that people are finding the subject matter a bit heavy, or something happens within the group which necessitates an additional short break. It is important that the trainer can be flexible and adapt to the needs of the group. Also, it should be the right of participants (not just the trainer) to request a break.

Some staff groups need to be put at ease by stating the obvious – 'you can get up and go to the toilet if the need arises'. I have come across many staff who have said they feel it is 'rude' to leave the room whilst the training is taking place and conse- quently have sat cross-legged until the break. This is not helpful as people become distracted; it is better that they get up and go when they have to! This is usually more of a problem during the afternoon, after numerous drinks have been consumed!

Ground rule 6: no mobile phones

This is a recent addition to my list of ground rules. During the past two years my training has been frequently interrupted by mobile phones ringing at the most inop- portune times. I now state that unless someone *has* to be on call, all mobile phones *must* be switched off.

The trainer should then ask participants to add their own ground rules in order to make them feel comfortable.

Programme

If there is a pool of trainers, then they must agree on a programme that they are going to follow, as there has to be consistency in the training provided. In the following chapter, some suggestions will be made regarding the content of basic rais- ing-awareness training.

Materials

The pool of trainers must also agree on the materials that are to be used in the training sessions – again to achieve consistency. Thought needs to be given to the design of handouts, overhead projections, case studies and exercises. All this needs to be prepared before the training sessions commence. The eventual objective will be to give each trainer a training pack. Suggestions for obtaining materials are made in the Appendix (page 170).

It cannot be emphasised enough that good preparation is crucial in order to provide effective training. From what has been discussed in this chapter, I hope it is clear that it is not enough for the trainer to just think about preparing him/herself. It is necessary to consider the needs of the participants and to anticipate situations that may arise during the training sessions (this will be discussed further in Chapters 6 and 7).

Endings

The pool of trainers must also reach some consensus about how they are going to wind down the group at the end of the course and how evaluations are going to be undertaken (which will be addressed in Chapter 8). If the course is only half a day, time will probably be very tight and trainers may prefer to have a quick ending so that most of the precious time can be used to deliver the content of the course. On longer courses it is important to:

- develop action plans
- obtain verbal and written evaluations about the course
- check that participants are emotionally OK
- give out attendance certificates.

Action plans

Participants may be very enthusiastic about a course and what they have learnt but as soon as they go back to the workplace much of the information may go to the back of their minds. They need to go away with a simple action plan which will act as trigger to remind them about what they need to do in the following three months.

DEVELOPING ACTION PLANS

Objective

For participants to develop a personal action plan to improve their practice in working with adult abuse.

Participants

Participants will work on their own.

Equipment

Prepared pro forma for action plan (see Handout 4.1).
Envelopes.

Time

5–10 minutes.

Task

Participants are asked to complete the action plan by thinking about:

• what they need to develop for their own good practice

• five tasks they are definitely going to undertake in the next three months.

After the plans have been completed, the trainer will give each participant an envelope in which to place the plan. On the envelope the participants will write 'Adult Abuse'. The trainer will ask participants to get out their diaries and turn to the date exactly *three months ahead*. They are asked to write in the diaries 'Open Adult Abuse Envelope'. Participants can look at the plan within the three-month period to remind themselves about their objectives, but on the 'opening day' they should review what they have achieved. If staff from the same workplace are attending a course together, they should agree to open the envelopes together.

Action plan

I, (Name of participant), promise myself that I will undertake the following in the next three months to improve my practice in adult abuse work:

A. *Subject areas to work on*

(List subject areas you are weak on or feel unsure about, i.e. consider what skills you need to develop.)

1.

2.

3.

B. *Tasks to be undertaken*

(Keep these tasks simple and achievable, e.g. re-reading the handouts from the course; taking an issue back to a manager/team.)

1.

2.

3.

4.

5.

Signed... Date....................

© Jacki Pritchard 2001

The emotional well-being of participants

It is very important that the trainer checks that everyone is feeling OK at the end of the course, i.e. not going home worrying about issues or going away upset, angry etc. An experienced trainer will usually pick up on the fact that someone is not OK and when this happens it is necessary to talk to the participant before s/he leaves. Some participants find it hard to admit that they are worried or having to deal with their emotions. So it can be useful to end with a small exercise (Exercise 4.2) which gives participants the opportunity to write down their feelings.

Attendance certificates

Nowadays most organisations have attendance certificates for courses (see example on page 68). This is very important when staff have personal development and training files or they are undertaking National Vocational Qualifications (NVQ). If a trainer is working independently, s/he can be asked to supply certificates, so these should be designed to show the following:

- title of course
- duration
- date
- venue
- learning outcomes
- NVQ modules
- trainer and trainer's qualifications.

HOW DO YOU FEEL?

Objective

To give participants the opportunity to tell the trainer they are not OK privately and not in a public forum.

Participants

To work on their own.

Equipment

Post-it stickers.

Time

1 minute.

Tasks for trainer

- Give post-it stickers to participants at the same time as they are given evaluation forms.

- Tell the group that if anyone is not OK and wants to talk privately after the course, they should indicate that.

- At the end of the course make approaches to people who have indicated they are not OK; they will be expecting this.

Task for participants

Participants are asked to write one word or one sentence about how they are feeling at the end of the course.

© Jacki Pritchard 2001

Certificate of Attendance

This is to certify that

(Insert name of participant)

attended a two-day training course

ADULT ABUSE: BASIC AWARENESS

on

(Insert date)

at

(Insert venue)

Learning outcomes

By the end of the course participants have:

- raised their awareness on the whole issue of adult abuse
- developed skills to be able to recognise signs and symptoms of adult abuse
- examined values and attitudes in regard to working with adult abuse
- an overview of legislation available
- a good working knowledge of what constitutes good practice
- more confidence in working with adult abuse.

This training will provide evidence of underpinning knowledge for NVQ Level 3 in Care in the following units and elements:

U4a10, U4b5, U4e1, U4e2, U4e3, U4e6, U4e7, W1d10, Z1c, Z18a, Z18b

Signed .... Date..............

Jacki Pritchard, Trainer
B.A. (HONS) in Economics; M.A. in Applied Social Studies
C.Q.S.W; CCETSW Practice Teaching Award.

Chapter 5

Content of a Basic Raising-awareness Course

This chapter will focus on the possible content of a basic raising-awareness course on adult abuse. I have stated in previous chapters that I believe that more advanced courses should be provided by 'an expert'; that is, someone who has had direct experience of working with abuse, been involved in investigations and undertaken long-term work with victims (and possibly abusers). It is important on advanced courses that the trainer can answer questions confidently and relate them to direct work experience. Participants are often critical if the trainer is detached from the real world. The trainer needs to have an understanding of the problems relating to practice.

Deciding on content

The content of the course will be decided either by the organisation or the pool of trainers who are going to provide the training. An organisation may have very set ideas at the outset about the content because of objectives they have developed previously. If this is the case, it is important for that organisation to state the purpose of the training programme (as discussed in Chapter 1), and course participants also need to be informed about this before attending a course. Otherwise, they may come with very different expectations.

Three basic questions need to be addressed on an awareness course:

- What is abuse?

- How do you recognise abuse?

- What do you do if you find or suspect abuse?

Consequently the course content should cover:

- Definitions of abuse

- Signs and symptoms

- Local policy and procedures.

The course content may be decided by people other than the trainers in the pool (training officer, independent consultant), who then have to be trained on how to present the information. Alternatively, the trainers may be able to design the course content themselves. If this is so, it is important that they have access to reading and training materials, so that they can develop their own knowledge but use materials they feel comfortable with. I am very conscious of the fact that trainers in a pool have limited time to read around a subject and will probably do this in their own time. They need to have easy access to materials and agencies should provide them with the basic texts. The 'Suggested Reading' list in the Appendix to this guide includes materials which I think are useful. There is now a substantial amount of literature on adult abuse, but not all of it is good and much is repetitive.

Trainers should try to read as much material as possible before attending sessions with other trainers in the pool, as they may have to spend time deciding what is going to be included on overheard slides (OHPs) and handouts; much time can be wasted during training-the-trainer sessions in undertaking this task. It is important that agreement is reached about handouts, overhead projections etc. so that there is consistency in the content of the courses which are to be provided. The trainers themselves will have different styles of presentation and that is fine, but the information given needs to be consistent.

When planning the sessions that are to be incorporated into a training course it is useful to think about what methods could be used. There needs to be a variety of methods to keep the participants interested (see Handout 5.1 on the next page). Also, getting them to work in pairs or small groups gets them to move physically, which is important. People lose concentration when they sit in the same place for any length of time. A variety of training methods needs to be used in order to keep a participant's attention. It is useful for a trainer to regularly remind him/herself of the following statistics. People remember:

- 10% of what they read
- 20% of what they hear
- 30% of what they see
- 50% of what they see and hear together
- 80% of what they say
- 90% of what they say while they do it

(NACRO Training and Development Services (1992) page 10)

Planning the content of the course could begin with Exercise 5.1 on page 73. Trainers need to become familiar with reading and training materials, but they also need to keep themselves up to date with developments in the adult abuse field. Two major requirements of any trainer will be to become familiar with:

- *No Secrets*, launched by the Department of Health in March 2000
- local policy and procedures.

Possible training methods

- Lecture/formal presentation

- Exercises – working as an individual or in small/large groups

- Group discussion

- Demonstration

- Video

- Quiz/games

- Questionnaires

- Role play

- Simulation

- Debates/panels

- Case studies

- Sculpting

- Art/drawing

PLANNING SESSIONS

Objective

To help participants decide which methods should be used for each part/session of the course.

Participants

This exercise can be undertaken in small groups or one large group, depending on how many trainers are in the pool.

Equipment

Copies of handout 5.1
Flipchart paper and pens

Time

30 minutes in small group for each section of the course.
Feedback: as long as it takes for a consensus to be reached within the pool.

Task

As each part of the course is being considered, participants are asked to answer the following question:

- What is the best possible way to present this information?

Feedback

Each group will feedback their ideas and then the pool as a whole will decide which methods will be adopted.

I have already stated what I believe should be the three main elements of any basic course on adult abuse, and the content will be partly dependent on how much time the trainer is given to deliver the course. On the facing page (p.75), I give some suggestions as to which subject areas should be included in individual sessions of a course (not all of which could be included if time is limited to half a day).

Definitions

A crucial part of any basic awareness course is defining adult abuse, and this is usually where the course starts. I have found that workers generally feel very uncomfortable about defining abuse and complain that 'there are too many grey areas'. I agree that this is an incredibly difficult area, because everyone has his/her own set of values and attitudes, which in turn may affect a personal definition of abuse. What may be seen as abusive behaviour to one person, may be acceptable behaviour to another. This is when conflict can develop between people – professionals, other workers, family members – even workers within the same organisation may have differing viewpoints.

In my training sessions I always emphasise that no-one can say you are right or you are wrong; it is open to interpretation. What is important is that participants think about the definition and by the end of the training course they are clear in their own minds both about what abuse means to them and the organisation's definition. The trainer must make clear what is expected of the worker in the job, or abuse may go unreported.

Very often people tend to think of abuse in terms of physical and sexual abuse. Therefore, it is important to get people thinking more broadly. This can be done in a number of ways. If time is limited, then the trainer may decide to have discussions in a large group using the flipchart to collate ideas and then relate to local definitions. If time is not tight, several exercises could be undertaken during this session (for examples see Pritchard 1996 – Chapter 1). Participants need to be led to think about:

- What does abuse mean to you personally?
- What does abuse mean to the organisation/local agencies?

This could be done by using Exercises 5.2 and 5.3 on pages 76 and 77.

- Historical perspective – developments in North America, the UK and locally

- Definitions

- Categories of abuse

- Who is a victim/who is an abuser? (i.e. focusing on the problem of stereotyping, discrimination, oppression etc)

- Where abuse happens

- Why abuse happens (presentation of different theories – causes/explanations)

- Statistics (national and local if available, to show prevalence)

- Institutional abuse

- Signs and symptoms

- Principles fundamental to working with abuse

- Ethics/confidentiality/sharing of information

- Policy/procedures

- Inter-agency working

- Roles of workers

- The law

WHAT IS ABUSE?

Objective

To make participants think about what constitutes abuse.

Participants

Exercise to be carried out in small groups.

Equipment

Flipchart paper and pens.

Time

Groups: 15 minutes to make lists.
Feedback: 30 minutes.

Task

Groups are asked to make two lists of definitions of abuse by thinking about:

• What abuse do you see/hear about when you are *not* at work?

• What abuse do you come across/hear about in your work situation?

Feedback

In large group.

WHAT DO I MEAN BY ABUSE?

Objective

To make participants think about what abuse means to them personally.

Participants

To work on their own.

Equipment

Large colourful post-it stickers (size 76mm x 127mm).

Time

Participants to make their own lists: 10 minutes.

The lists are then stuck on a wall and read: 5 minutes.

Feedback: 15 minutes.

Task

Participants are asked to list their own definitions of abuse. This can be done in very simple terms, e.g. acts and behaviour.

Feedback

Large group discussion.

After exercises have been undertaken to stimulate discussion, the trainer needs to link the discussion that has taken place to national and local definitions. Handouts/OHPs should have been designed to help the presentation. It is helpful to focus the discussion on:

1. **Definitions of adult abuse** – national and local (For examples, see Handouts 5.2 and 5.3 on pages 79 and 80.)

2. **Categories of abuse** – giving examples of what comes under each heading. This should be linked closely to what is in the local policy procedure. (For examples see Handouts 5.3, 5.4 and 5.5 on pages 80, 81 and 82.)

Handout 5.5 is an example of how the key parts from a document can be presented concisely rather than participants having to wade through a policy document during a course. In Wakefield Metropolitan District Council's policy and procedure document *Adult Abuse and Protection* the categories of abuse were presented together with indicators over four pages. For training purposes the key definitions were summarised and quoted on one side of A4 paper.

The trainer should not bombard participants with too much information early on in the course. It is good to break into groups for the exercises suggested above or to discuss specific issues or dilemmas.

TOPICS FOR DISCUSSION

- Should stranger abuse be included in definitions of adult abuse?

- Should self-neglect be included in definitions of abuse?

- Do we hide behind the principle of choice when dealing with self-neglect?

- Why is adult abuse a form of domestic violence?

- Who comes under the brief of domestic violence organisations?

The systematic maltreatment, physical, emotional or financial, of an elderly person... this may take the form of physical assault, threatening behaviour, neglect, abandonment or sexual assault.

(From: page 3, Eastman, M. (1984) *Old Age abuse.*
London: Age Concern)

Abuse may be described as physical, sexual, psychological or financial. It may be intentional or unintentional, or the result of neglect. It causes harm to the older person, either temporarily or over a period of time.

(From: page 3, Department of Health (1993) *No longer afraid: the safeguard of older people in domestic settings.* London: HMSO)

Elder abuse is a single or repeated act or lack of appropriate action occurring within any relationship where there is an expectation of trust which causes harm or distress to an older person.

(From: Action on Elder Abuse Bulletin, No 11,
(1995) London: AEA)

...a violation of an individual's human and civil rights by any other person or persons.

(From: page 9, Department of Health (2000)
No Secrets. London: HMSO)

Key definitions from No Secrets

A vulnerable adult is a person:

"who is or may be in need of community care services by reason of mental or other disability, age or illness; and who is or may be unable to take care of him or herself, or unable to protect him or herself against significant harm or exploitation".

(From: Green Paper Who Decides? *London: Lord Chancellor's Department 1997)*

Abuse is:

"a violation of an individual's human and civil rights by any other person or persons"

Forms of abuse:

- Physical abuse

- Sexual abuse

- Psychological abuse

- Financial or material

- Neglect and acts of omission

- Discriminatory abuse

From: Department of Health (2000) *No Secrets.* London: HMSO

Categories of adult abuse

PHYSICAL

EMOTIONAL/PSYCHOLOGICAL

FINANCIAL

NEGLECT

SEXUAL

Local definitions of abuse

Physical

This includes falls or injuries which are not satisfactorily explained, or, where the explanation offered is not conducive to the present injuries. It also includes rough handling or the use of restraint.

Emotional/psychological

Fear through threats of force, intimidation, humiliation or emotional blackmail which can include socially isolating the individual, or denying them choice, e.g. through preventing them receiving services.

Financial

The denial of access of the individual to money, property and possessions, through acts of omission or commission, or the extortion of such through threats.

Neglect

The withholding of adequate care for daily living to the individual, whether intentional or unintentional. This includes nutrition, treatments, or administering an inappropriate level of treatment. It also involves non-intervention to prevent harm to an individual who is not considered to have sufficient capacity to appreciate risk.

Sexual

The involvement of adults in sexual activities without their informed consent, or where the individual has insufficient mental capacity to have full understanding of the activity. This relates to all forms of sexual activity including non contact activity such as pornography, voyeurism and exhibitionism.

(From: Wakefield Housing and Social Care (1999) *Adult Abuse and Protection: Policy and Procedures*. Wakefield: Metropolitan District Council)

Institutional abuse needs to be mentioned in definitions, but if time allows, it is better to address this subject in a longer session later in the course. *No Secrets* does highlight the need to address institutional abuse:

> 2.9 Neglect and poor professional practice also need to be taken into account. This may take the form of isolated incidents of poor or unsatisfactory professional practice, at one end of the spectrum, through to pervasive ill treatment or gross misconduct at the other. Repeated instances of poor care may be an indication of more serious problems and this is sometimes referred to as **institutional abuse**.
>
> (p.10, DOH 2000)

Participants need to be encouraged to talk about cultures of care and the more subtle forms of abuse. This is especially important for staff working in residential/day care and hospital settings. Ready-made exercises and materials are presented in *Working with Elder Abuse: A Training Manual for Home Care, Residential and Day Care Staff* (Pritchard 1996) and can be adapted for awareness training on adult abuse courses.

Signs and symptoms

It takes time to learn how to recognise abuse, and workers become more confident with experience in the field. However, the majority of workers are not specialising in adult abuse and may only deal with such cases from time to time. It is hard to learn indicators of abuse and retain that information if it is not being used on a daily basis. This is a difficult area in which to teach and train workers; and sometimes the information can be overwhelming for course participants. When planning a course, trainers need to give a great deal of thought to *how* the information is going to be presented. Trainers need to ensure that they are confident themselves in having this knowledge before they begin training in this area. If the trainer has not had a great deal of experience in identifying abuse then it is crucial that s/he spends time learning the signs and symptoms, but s/he also has to acquire the knowledge about indicators which can be the symptom of something else.

Many policy and procedure documents follow similar formats now, and most include signs and indicators of abuse. Again it is important that trainers link the training to what is printed in the document and produce handouts which are easy to understand and grasp, rather than reprinting the document word for word. Handouts 5.6 to 5.10 on pages 85–89 give some simplified examples (from Chapter 2, Pritchard 1996), but it is also useful to refer to Appendix 1 in *No Longer Afraid*, which summarises the indicators of abuse; the various tables could be reproduced as OHPs or handouts (DOH 1993). There are certain points that the trainer must emphasise to the participants. Some trainers prefer not to go through lists, but to facilitate learning by introducing case studies or short vignettes as shown in Exercise 5.4 (p.90).

TRAINER TIPS: KEY POINTS TO EMPHASISE

- Abuse can be extremely difficult to recognise.

- Abuse often remains well hidden (for a variety of reasons).

- It can take years to identify or prove that abuse has taken place.

- The victim may deny that abuse is happening to protect the abuser.

- Many victims will choose to remain in the abusive situation.

- Many signs of abuse can be indicators of other things; therefore, one should not jump to conclusions but keep an open mind.

- It is important to monitor changes in behaviour over time (use Handout 5.10 to emphasise this).

- It is often people who know the victim well who will notice the gradual changes in behaviour.

- Workers should not feel guilty if they 'miss' signs of abuse (especially when thinking back to past cases).

Physical indications of abuse
(this includes physical neglect)

- Multiple bruising, not consistent with a fall.

- Black eyes, slap marks, kick marks, other bruises.

- Burns, not consistent with scorching by direct heat.

- Fractures not consistent with falls.

- Stench of urine or faeces.

- Indications of malnutrition or over-feeding.

- Absence of mobility aids.

- Administration of inappropriate drugs or the absence of necessary medication.

© Jacki Pritchard 1996

Indicators of sexual abuse

- Genital or urinary irritation.

- Frequent infections (evidence of vaginal discharge may be found on knickers).

- Bleeding (blood can be found on underwear, nightclothes).

- Sexually transmitted disease.

- Bruising on inner thighs.

- Difficulty in walking/sitting.

- Sudden onset of confusion.

- Depression.

- Nightmares.

- Severe upset or agitation when the older person is being bathed, dressed, undressed, or medically examined (or when these things are suggested).

- Conversation regularly becomes of a sexual nature.

Indicators of emotional abuse
(this includes emotional neglect)

- Insomnia/deprivation of sleep or need for excessive sleep.

- Change in appetite.

- Unusual weight gain/loss.

- Weepiness/unusual bouts of sobbing/crying.

- Unexplained paranoia.

- Low self esteem.

- Excessive fear/anxiety.

- Ambivalence.

Indicators of financial abuse

- Unexplained or sudden inability to pay bills (e.g. rent, gas, electricity, no money for food/shopping).

- Unexplained or sudden withdrawal of money from post office/bank/building society accounts.

- Disparity between assets and satisfactory living conditions.

- Lack of receptivity by the older person or relative/neighbour to any necessary assistance requiring expenditure, when finances are not a problem.

- Extraordinary interest by family members and other people in the older person's assets/will.

Known reactions to abuse

- The denial (often forthright) that anything is amiss, with an accompanying emphasis that things 'have never been better'.

- Resignation, stoicism, and, sometimes, an acceptance of incidents as being part of being old/vulnerable.

- Withdrawal from activity, communication and participation.

- Marked change in behaviour and inappropriate attachments. Fear, subsequently combined with depression and a sense of hopelessness.

- Mental confusion.

- Anger and physical/verbal outbursts.

- Seeking attention/protection, often from numerous sources (some of which can be unlikely).

SPOT THE ABUSE

Objective

To help participants identify signs of abuse and to categorise abuse.

Participants

Exercise to be carried out in small groups.

Equipment

Flipchart paper and pens.

Case studies which have been prepared beforehand. Trainers need to have developed enough case studies to ensure that they illustrate different client groups, a variety of indicators and types of abuse. Sometimes it is better to have short vignettes. Some material is presented as case studies in Chapter 9.

Time

Group work: 20 minutes to study vignettes.
Feedback: 30–40 minutes.

Task

Groups are asked to study the vignettes and list the indicators of abuse in each one. They also need to state which category(ies) of abuse they think are taking place.

Policy and procedure

This is always the difficult bit, because many workers are 'turned off' by policy documents. It is difficult for the trainer too; it is necessary to try to make the session as interesting as possible because it is crucial that participants go away from the course knowing what they are expected to do if they find or suspect abuse. Some trainers I know do prefer to go through the relevant part of the document page by page. I personally find this tedious and boring. I think it is necessary to design a simple handout which gets across the stages of the process. Some documents will have flowcharts and again these can be useful as handouts (see pages 92–94).

Some organisations have small leaflets which are produced for staff as an 'easy guide' (see example on page 95–96). Larger agencies may produce leaflets which are to be circulated at the time of launching a new policy and are distributed internally and within the local area (e.g. libraries, recreation centres).

The trainer must get across the following points:

KEY POINTS TO EMPHASISE

- When to report abuse.
- Who to report to, i.e. line manager, other points of referral.
- Who will be responsible for investigating.
- Timescales.
- The process, i.e. moving through referral/allegation/suspicion, investigation, case conference, development of protection plan, review.
- The different agencies/people who could be involved.
- Potential roles of workers who are present on the course.
- Distinguish between the short- and long-term work.

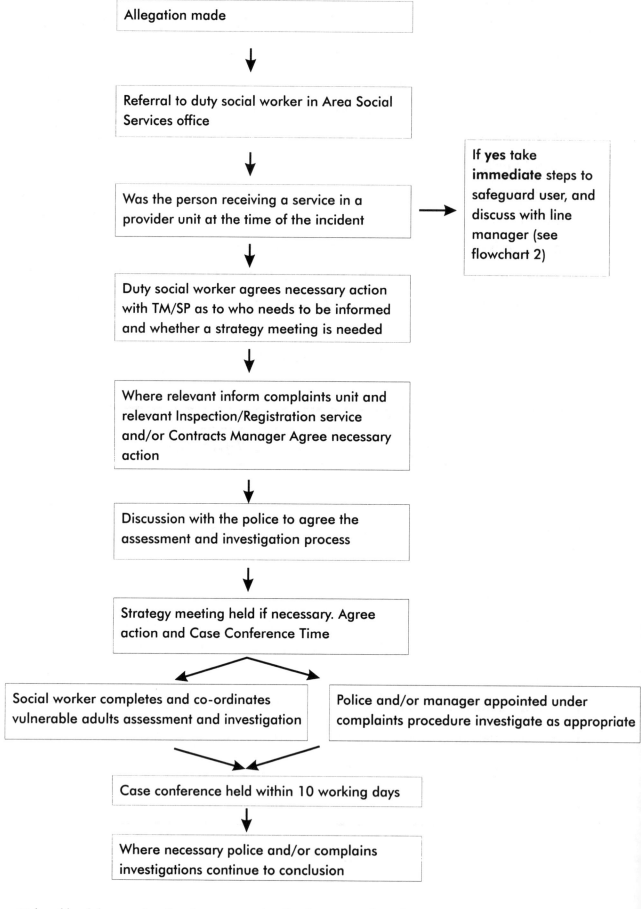

Allegation made

↓

Referral to duty social worker in Area Social Services office

↓

Was the person receiving a service in a provider unit at the time of the incident → If **yes** take **immediate** steps to safeguard user, and discuss with line manager (see flowchart 2)

↓

Duty social worker agrees necessary action with TM/SP as to who needs to be informed and whether a strategy meeting is needed

↓

Where relevant inform complaints unit and relevant Inspection/Registration service and/or Contracts Manager Agree necessary action

↓

Discussion with the police to agree the assessment and investigation process

↓

Strategy meeting held if necessary. Agree action and Case Conference Time

↙   ↘

Social worker completes and co-ordinates vulnerable adults assessment and investigation   Police and/or manager appointed under complaints procedure investigate as appropriate

↘   ↙

Case conference held within 10 working days

↓

Where necessary police and/or complains investigations continue to conclusion

Vulnerable adults procedure flowchart. From: City of Stoke on Trent (1999) Policy and Procedure for the Protection of Vulnerable Adults (Including Interagency Guidelines).

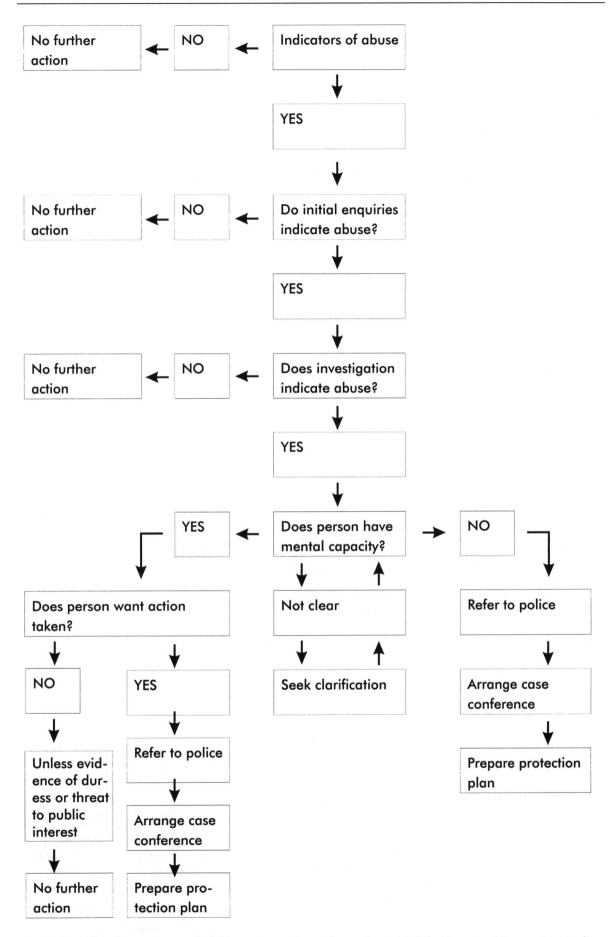

Investigation flowchart. From: Wakefield Housing and Social Care (1999) Adult Abuse and Protection: Policy and Procedures. *Wakefield: Metropolitan District Council.*

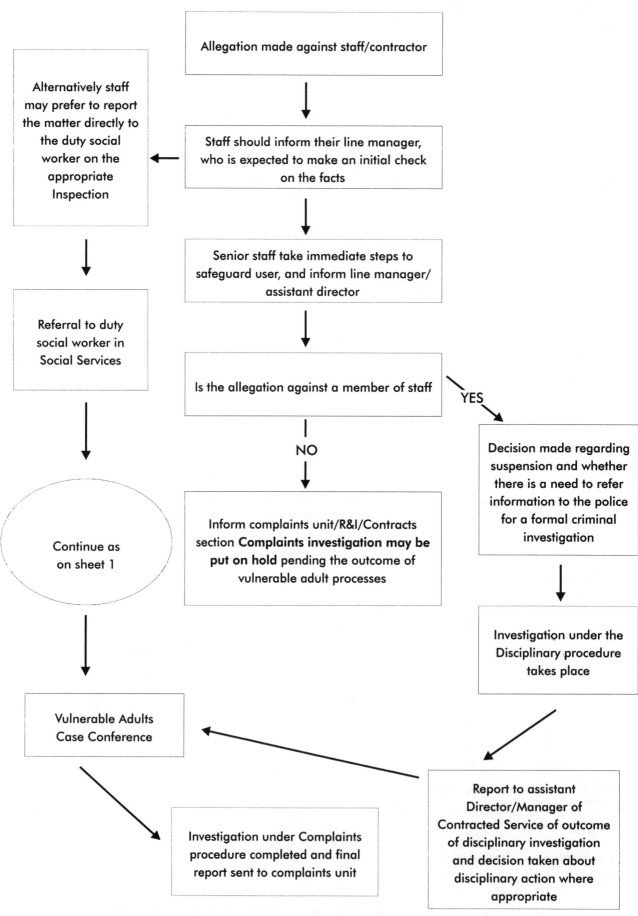

Vulnerable adults procedure flowchart 2. From: City of Stoke on Trent (1999) Policy and Procedure for the Protection of Vulnerable Adults (Including Interagency Guidelines).

Q&A

Q What is abuse?

A Abuse is where harm is caused, deliberately or not, to another individual. It might be because someone is hit, sexually interfered with, or the victim of theft. It can also be intentional, unintentional, or the result of neglect.

Q Where does it happen?

A Anywhere! It can happen in people's own homes, in residential or nursing homes, in day centres or in hospital.

Q How will I know abuse is going on?

A The full document gives a complete picture, but here are some indicators to look for:

- **unexplained injuries or falls**
- **frequent visits to the doctor or A & E**
- **bruises**
- **weight loss**
- **mood swings**
- **pressure sores or ulcers**

3

Contents

Introduction

This leaflet is a brief summary of the Adult Abuse and Protection, Policy and Procedures which addresses the issue of abuse of vulnerable adults.

This guide is intended only as an overview to help staff in the first instance.

The full document explains in more detail the issues surrounding the abuse of vulnerable adults and is essential reading.

Reading this leaflet should help you:

- **recognise abuse**
- **know who to talk to about it**

2

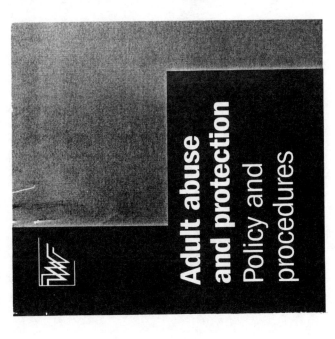

Adult abuse and protection
Policy and procedures

An introductory summary for staff

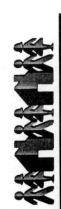

Housing & Social Care

Working together for better communities

95

- **isolation**
- **fear**
- **lack of money**

Q Who can I talk to?

A Talk to your supervisor. They will arrange for the situation to be carefully looked at. Your contribution will be very important.

Q What about confidentiality?

A Discuss this with your supervisor. Sometimes people do not want things to change and their view should be respected. Your supervisor will ask for advice as well.

Our commitment to you

All staff have responsibility to report all concerns regarding abuse or suspected abuse. Staff have the right to expect that their concerns are acted upon and treated seriously.

If you think your supervisor is not taking the right action then talk to *their* manager! When you do speak out you will be supported and action will not be taken against you.

Useful telephone contacts

The five Community Care teams are:

1 **Community Care Team** *Ferry Fryston Base*
01977 722125
890 2125 (internal)
Children's Team *Normanton Base*
01924 302400
850 2400 (internal)

2 **Community Care Team** *Featherstone Base*
01977 722640
890 2640 (internal)
Children's Team *Featherstone Base*
01977 722640
890 2640 (internal)

3 **Community Care Team** *South Elmsall Base*
01977 723245
890 2345 (internal)
Children's Team *Hemsworth Base*
01977 722305
890 2305 (internal)

4 **Community Care Team** *Portobello Base*
01924 303260
850 3260 (internal)
Children's Team *Ossett Base*
01924 303000
850 3000 (internal)

5 **Community Care Team** *Flanshaw Base*
01924 302195
850 2195 (internal)
Children's Team *Eastmoor Base*
01924 302615
850 2615 (internal)

Relevant circulars

C18/1999 Adult Abuse and Protection, Policy and Procedures
C15/1997 The Disciplinary Procedure
C18/1996 The Complaint's procedure
C6/1998 Appropriate Boundaries
P6/1996 Whistle Blowing
C1/1997 Employee Code of Conduct

Wakefield MDC
Housing & Social Care
8 St. John's North, Wakefield WF1 3QA
T. 01924 307700 F. 01924 307792

Ref 34864. Designed by WMDC Design & Print Services. 01924 305776

Most organisations will have a monitoring form that has to be completed if they work on an adult abuse referral and/or investigation. The trainer needs to explain clearly what is expected of workers regarding the established monitoring systems. Monitoring forms often prove to be problematic because workers are unsure when to complete them.

It is important during this session that the trainer talks about:

- Values and principles underpinning adult abuse work.

- What constitutes good practice.

It is usually at this point that questions come hard and fast from participants and trainers should leave adequate time when planning this part of the course to allow a full discussion to take place. Anxieties frequently centre around issues regarding the sharing of information and breaking confidentiality. Handouts 5.11 and 5.12 (pages 98 and 99) can be used to facilitate discussion if necessary.

It is at this point that the trainer needs to allow plenty of time for discussion, because it will be at this time that workers will be questioning their own role and getting anxious about what they might have to do. Some typical questions which might be put to the trainer are:

- Will I have to be involved in investigations/interviewing?

- Will I have to deal with the alleged abuser?

- Will I have to attend a case conference?

- Will I have to talk to the police?

- Whose responsibility is it to inform the police about the case/or ask for a joint investigation?

- What if I have missed abuse and someone else spots it? Will I be disciplined?

- What if you can't get the right people to come to the case conference within the time limit?

- What if I don't follow the procedure exactly? Will I be in trouble?

- Who can I share information with?

- What if the victim doesn't want to do anything about the abuse?

PRINCIPLES OF ADULT ABUSE WORK

SELF DETERMINATION

CONFIDENTIALITY

DIGNITY

CHOICE

EQUAL OPPORTUNITIES

GOOD PRACTICE

In order to promote good practice it is necessary to remember the following:

- The welfare of the victim is of paramount importance.

- The victim has rights, e.g. to self determination.

- You are dealing with adults not children.

- You must report any suspicion/allegation of abuse to your line manager.

- You must not keep concerns/worries to yourself.

- You are bound by confidentiality, but in some circumstances this has to be broken.

- You must listen to the victim.

- Do not jump to conclusions before you have all the facts, i.e. do not write the script.

- Do not be tempted to stereotype victims and abusers.

- Do not dismiss a disclosure of abuse from someone who does not have full mental capacity.

- Do not be judgemental.

- Observe what is happening to your service user.

- Never panic/keep calm.

- Do not show shock or horror.

- Talk about how you are feeling to your manager.

The law

Participants attending a basic awareness course on adult abuse do not need to be bombarded with information about the law. They will probably be struggling enough to take in all the information about what constitutes abuse and recognising abuse. However, the trainer does need to address the law in some way, because many workers may come with the pre-conceived idea that because there is no statutory framework as such for adult abuse, nothing can be done legally to help a victim. It is true that legal provision is poor and needs to be developed, but the trainer needs to emphasise that the criminal justice system can be used positively in some cases and sometimes civil law can also be utilised. Again, it is vital to emphasise the importance of inter-agency working and the role of the police, who can respond sensitively to adult abuse cases.

Most local policy and procedure documents incorporate a section on the legal framework. It is helpful to alert course participants to this and suggest to them that they read it in depth at a later date. It may be useful to have a handout which summarises the key statutes as in Handout 5.13 (page 101), which participants can use as a reference point in the future. I believe that the law needs to be addressed in depth either in a more advanced course (like investigation) or in a specific module when a legal expert could be brought in. However, on a basic raising-awareness course the following should be mentioned:

TRAINER TIPS: KEY POINTS TO EMPHASISE

- The location of the legal section in the local policy and procedure document.

- Dilemmas – assessing mental capacity and the right to self determination.

- Specific legislation that could be used in adult abuse cases e.g. Mental Health Act 1983, Family Law Act 1996, Harassment Act 1997.

- The issue of confidentiality and the sharing of information relating this to the Crime and Disorder Act 1998 – particularly Section 115 (regarding the sharing information principle).

Relevant Legislation

- Civil Evidence Act 1968

- Crime and Disorder Act 1998

- Criminal Law Act 1967

- Enduring Powers of Attorney Act 1985

- Family Law Act 1996 (Part IV)

- Housing Act 1996 (Part VII)

- Human Rights Act 1998

- Mental Health Act 1983

- National Assistance Act 1948 – Section 47

- NHS and Community Care Act 1990

- Police and Criminal Evidence Act 1984

- Power of Attorney Act 1971

- Protection from Harassment Act 1997

- Registered Homes Act 1984

- Sexual Offences Act 1956

- Torts (Inteference with Goods) Act 1977

Although the basic raising-awareness course will not go into great detail about the law, the trainer does need to have read/be familiar with *Speaking Up For Justice* (Home Office 1998) and *Action for Justice* (Home Office March 1999), which are concerned with vulnerable adults or intimidated witnesses in the criminal justice system.

Endings

Trainers will need to think about how they are going to end a course and this will be addressed in Chapter 9.

References

City of Stoke On Trent (1999) *Policy and Procedure For the Protection of Vulnerable Adults (including Inter-Agency Guidelines)*. Stoke On Trent: City of Stoke On Trent.

Department of Health (1993) *No Longer Afraid: The Safeguard of Older People in Domestic Settings*. London: HMSO.

Department of Health (2000) *No Secrets: guidance on developing and implementing multi-agency policies and procedures to protect vulnerable adults from abuse*. London: HMSO.

Eastman, M. (1984) *Old Age Abuse*. London: Age Concern.

Home Office (March 1999) *Action for Justice*. London: HMSO.

Home Office (1998) *Speaking Up For Justice*. London HMSO.

NACRO Training and Development Services (1992) *A Guide to Good Practice in Training*. London: NACRO.

Pritchard, J. (1996) *Working with Elder Abuse: A Training Manual for Home Care, Residential and Day Care Staff*. London: Jessica Kingsley Publishers.

Wakefield Housing and Social Care (1999) *Adult Abuse and Protection: Policy and Procedures*. Wakefield: Metropolitan District Council.

Wakefield Housing and Social Care (1999) *Adult Abuse and Protection: Policy and Procedures: An Introductory Summary for Staff*. Wakefield: Metropolitan District Council.

Chapter 6

Difficult Issues for the Trainer

In this chapter I want to discuss some of the more difficult issues a trainer may face when actually running a course. These are:

- breaking confidentiality
- participants not being able to cope with the subject of abuse
- handling disclosure from course participants
- reporting abusive or bad practice.

People who are new to training probably do not want to hear any of this because they have got enough to think about in providing the course; nevertheless, they are issues which must be faced and addressed.

Confidentiality

As was discussed in Chapter 4 the trainer must deal with the issue of confidentiality at the beginning of any course (Ground rule 3 – see Chapter 4). On most courses there will not be a problem. Participants will learn to trust each other and usually be willing to engage in full discussions about work practices and the service users they work with. It is only when difficult issues arise, such as will be discussed below, that confidentiality will have to be broken. It is important for trainers to realise that situations are going to arise where confidentiality must be broken in the interest of promoting good practice and safeguarding service users.

Not coping with the subject of abuse

In earlier chapters I referred to the fact that participants can be greatly affected by the content of an abuse course and it is crucial that a trainer is able to pick up on the signs that someone may be distressed and to offer the appropriate support. When working in the social care field the term 'abuse' is used frequently and we know that abuse is very prevalent. Society in general has now accepted that child abuse does occur across the social classes, whereas 20 years ago it was still a taboo subject; similarly, people have become more aware of domestic violence. People cannot fail to hear about abuse when in recent years the media has sensationalised such horrific cases as Rikki Neave, the victims of Fred and Rosemary West, institutional abuse in North Wales etc. However, adult abuse does not get such a high profile so participants on a course may be 'quite shocked'.

For those of us who are working with abuse every day of our lives, we might get a bit blasé about it (although we would never admit it!); that is, we are not easily shocked. In order to cope we have developed strategies (as victims of abuse do) and may have 'hardened up' in the sense that we are able to deal effectively with the different emotions which can be evoked when dealing with abuse cases. For others who are not dealing with abuse regularly the emotions can be difficult to cope with. I am often asked when training: 'How do you cope with dealing with abuse cases all the time?'; 'How do you cut off when you get home?': 'Does it affect you?' 'How do you sleep at night?'.

I believe that not everyone is able to work with abuse; we are all good at different things and may develop specialised skills to deal with particular problems or service user groups. When working with abuse in particular I think it is crucial to develop specific coping strategies, so that you can vent your feelings appropriately (and there will be a whole range of emotions to experience when dealing with cases of abuse) and that you are able to cut off once away from work. I think it is important to have interests and leisure activities outside of work that are not related to the job at all. I think it also helps to have friends who are not in the social care field too so that you are not talking about 'the job' all the time.

When working in the field of abuse it can be easy to forget that abuse is not a daily topic of conversation for other people; a vast number of people never have to think about abuse at all in the normal course of their lives. So to come on a training course and to have to learn about what constitutes abuse can be extremely upsetting for some people, especially if they tend to look for the good in people.

Trainers may have to deal with responses they would not normally expect to hear. For example, I find that home care and residential staff often verbalise their gut reaction and are totally honest about how they feel:

'I'd cut his bloody balls off.'

'He should be put away for life.'

> (Home carers' responses when discussing a case of incest between demented mother and son).

Inexperienced trainers will be concentrating hard on presenting information and getting the audience engaged and involved. An additional task is to watch participants very carefully and to observe closely their reactions. As shown above, some participants will openly verbalise their reactions; others may show emotion through their facial expressions; others will show how uncomfortable they are through their body language. So there is a great deal for the trainer to watch for and then decide how to deal with situations appropriately. As a trainer becomes more experienced s/he will pick up more easily the signs that someone is affected by the subject matter. This is also another good reason for having two trainers presenting the course. Whilst one trainer is leading/presenting, the other one will be observing the participants whilst also supporting his/her colleague.

The signs

So what are the signs that someone is not OK? Again, like victims, everyone reacts differently. Table 6.1 lists some of the typical reactions I see on a day-to-day basis.

Table 6.1 Typical Reactions

- Shock
- Horror
- Disbelief
- Sadness
- Upset/crying
- Anger
- Feeling sick

At the beginning of the course, it is important to watch the participants closely when stating the ground rules. A trainer must learn to look for reactions to what is said about acknowledging that some participants may find the subject area difficult and allowing them space (Ground rule 1 – see Chapter 4). Participants may suddenly:

- change their facial expressions

- go white/colour drains from face

- start fidgeting/fiddling

- look upset/burst into tears

- avoid the eyes of the trainer

- look at the floor

- look uncomfortable

- show a sign of relief.

The trainer then needs to watch carefully as the course proceeds. The signs that someone is not OK (as stated above) may show at any time during the course. In addition participants can:

- be overtly aggressive

- be confrontational

- go into denial

- be tearful

- withdraw/not participate.

TRAINER TIP

If you pick up that someone is feeling uncomfortable or their behaviour becomes unacceptable, then deal with the situation as soon as possible. Do not let it drag on.

Handling disclosure

We know that much abuse remains hidden and consequently we are unsure about the true prevalence of abuse within our society. It is probably much higher than research statistics indicate due to the fact that many victims are not known to any agencies. Trainers must be aware that some course participants will have experienced abuse themselves (in childhood and/or adulthood), some may still be living in abusive situations or they may be having to deal with a family member who is/or has been abused. Therefore, having to attend a course on abuse can be abusive in itself; but many organisations now make courses mandatory, so it is hard to avoid attendance.

Managers should be sensitive to the fact that workers may be at a stage in their life when it is not appropriate to attend a training course on abuse, because of any of the reasons stated above. There will be situations where the participant attends the course thinking they will be able to cope or where the participant has not disclosed any personal matters to the manager and has been sent to do the course because it is mandatory. Once on the course the participant may not be able to cope with the situation. The trainer has to support the participant through this and maybe make the decision *with* the participant not to continue at this particular time. Time will need to be spent with the participant to discuss their difficulties and a decision will have to be made regarding explanation to their line manager.

How often does disclosure happen?

When I am training a pool of trainers and I introduce the topic of having to handle disclosure, most people's faces drop and then I am asked about how frequently this occurs. It is important for me not to raise potential trainers' anxieties. I think it happens more frequently to trainers who are experienced in working abuse and who openly explain their work backgrounds and share their knowledge and experiences. In some ways giving this information is a way of 'giving permission to speak'. This is a concept I have discussed fully elsewhere in relation to working with victims of abuse (Pritchard 2000). If victims know that a person is knowledgeable in working with people who have been abused, they assume that person is unlikely to react adversely to hearing a disclosure about abuse and this facilitates disclosure from the victim. Many victims, whether children or adults, do not disclose about abuse because they fear they will not be believed, they will be laughed at, or the recipient will be shocked or upset by what s/he hears. Participants who are victims themselves will react in a similar way if they know the trainer has the necessary knowledge and experience. Because of the way they present themselves, some trainers will never be the recipients of disclosure. Their style or manner will prohibit victims from feeling safe to disclose. Another barrier to disclosure can be the fact that the trainer is from within the organisation, so may not been seen as a 'safe' person to talk to.

When and where does disclosure happen?

Disclosure is less likely to happen when the course is short in length (maybe only half a day), because much of the information given will not be in any great depth. Participants are more likely to be affected when the trainers go into more specific detail and there is in-depth discussion about actual cases or case studies, which brings reality to the session. While trainers talk about theory, it is easier for participants to detach themselves.

Handling a disclosure from a participant on a training course can be similar to receiving a disclosure when you are working closely with a victim in a work setting. I find myself handling disclosures from both workers and service users regularly through my working week and am constantly reminded about the similarities. For a trainer who is not experienced in receiving disclosure it would be worth reading my previous work on this subject (Chapter 4, Pritchard 1996).

The reality of training is that a disclosure can come at anytime and often it is when you least expect it (very much like a victim who discloses to someone when they are engaged in an intimate activity like toiletting or bathing). Some participants will disclose in the large group setting; this is more likely when participants have gelled together and some trust has been formed between them. Disclosure Example 1 is an example where the disclosure was very dramatic and had an adverse effect on the group.

In situations where a participant gives a disclosure to the group, the trainer needs to watch the rest of the group to see if they are comfortable with this and if so allow the disclosure to happen. A difficult task is judging how to manage the time. The disclosee needs time to vent, but the trainer is always worried about picking up the aftermath and how this will affect the agenda and timing of the course. Sometimes it will be necessary to stop the disclosure (as in Disclosure Example 1) or to give it a limited amount time and offer to pursue this with the disclosee at break time. It is a difficult judgement to make, but again comes with experience.

Disclosure Example I

The scenario

A social worker stood up in the middle of a session. She rolled her sleeves up very slowly and dramatically and then said 'This is what my father did to me'. She proceeded to show the group her scars from cigarette burns and cuts inflicted by a knife. She was very angry.

Effect on group

The majority were embarassed by her behaviour and shocked by the extent of the injuries which had been inflicted. It was obvious they felt uncomfortable and did not how to react.

Action

I made the decision to take the disclosee out of the room. Once I had got her into a quiet room, I went back to the group to set them an exercise whilst I dealt with the worker. After doing the exercise with the group I discussed with them what had happened and how they felt.

As stated previously, it is preferable to co-train and this helps to deal with difficult situations when they arise; or if you are training alone there should be someone else around (like a training officer) who can come in if there is a crisis. If there are two trainers, one can deal with the disclosee whilst the other trainer carries on with the course. If you are training alone, then you have to react to the presenting situation as best you can. In the example given above, the training officer had agreed to be around so she supervised the exercise I had given the group whilst I dealt with the disclosee.

Some people disclose in the group and are absolutely fine when they do this; they do not need to go out of the group for space. However, it is still very important for the trainer to follow-up at break time or after the course to check that the person is OK. Other disclosees are not OK at all and this needs to be dealt with immediately. They may need to leave the group during or after the disclosure. They will need to talk through their emotions and reactions; everything should be done to make sure they can leave feeling OK about what has happened. Sometimes it is not appropriate for the person to carry on with the course on that particular day.

TRAINER TIP

When planning a course, do not make timings too rigid. Allow for the fact that exercises and discussions could take longer than they should. Also disclosures and discussions about specific cases could cause delays. Therefore, there needs to be some flexibility.

Alternatively, if a participant has taken advantage of Ground rule 1 (space) and left the group, s/he may disclose to the trainer who comes to check if s/he is OK. It is important that the trainer does not intrude on this privacy by asking too many questions; the participant's welfare is the prime concern. The trainer needs to ask if the participant requires anything in particular to help the situation. Some will take this opportunity to disclose.

In other situations, a participant may disclose to the trainer during a break or at lunch time. The trainer can find him/herself under pressure because s/he will be conscious of when the next session is due to start. There is often a dilemma about suggesting to the participant that you will talk to them at a more appropriate time, because there is the possibility that the participant will choose not to continue if s/he cannot do it immediately. Once the participant starts talking, s/he will forget the time and again the trainer may feel rude if they have to terminate the discussion. Again, this is why it can be helpful to have two trainers presenting the session, so the trainer who receives the disclosure can remain with the disclosee.

I have often found that many people choose to disclose at the very end of the course. Perhaps this is because they feel safe telling someone whom they will not see again or because they feel they can escape quickly. This can be difficult for the trainer who is probably feeling very tired at the end of the course and may not have a lot left to give emotionally. It can also be quite damaging to the trainer when someone discloses and then that person makes it clear that s/he wishes to leave immediately rather than talking it through. Some people just have the need 'to tell' rather than discuss in depth. In these situations the trainer may be left with unresolved issues, i.e. the excess baggage, which is extremely uncomfortable and unsatisfactory.

Role of the trainer

The trainer's role is to *listen* to the disclosure; s/he should not try to get into a type of counselling role as time will not allow this and more harm than good could be done. It may be possible for the trainer to offer practical advice. The trainer should be assessing during the disclosure whether some sort of referral is needed. By 'referral' I mean whether the person needs further support from someone else. In some situations the trainer may decide that it is necessary to suggest that a line manager or training officer should be informed.

Sharing information and referring on

As well as ensuring that the person is all right on that day, the trainer must think about the aftermath and whether further support may be needed. In some circumstances it will be necessary to discuss with the participant whether information should be shared, e.g. the trainer may feel that in some circumstances the line manager or training officer needs to be informed because s/he has concerns about the participant's future well-being, but also there may be issues regarding the effect on the participant's work or work practices. Obviously, confidentiality must be maintained whenever possible, but in certain circumstances it will have to be broken.

TRAINER TIP

Do not get too involved when handling a disclosure and supporting the disclosee. Remember to:

- Listen

- Assess

- Advise

- Refer on if appropriate.

Disclosure Example 2

Disclosure

The participant, who is an unqualified social worker, disclosed that he had been a victim of physical abuse in childhood; this had involved extreme violence from his father. The basic raising-awareness course on adult abuse had triggered all sorts of memories for this man and he realised that he was still very angry towards his father and would find it difficult to work with anyone who perpetrated violence.

Action

The trainer suggested that the worker should explain his fears to his manager. The worker was reluctant to do this because he thought the male manager would see him 'as a wimp'. With the permission of the worker, the trainer agreed to contact the manager in the first instance to alert him to the situation. The manager agreed to meet with both the worker and the trainer.

The following checklist is a helpful tool to memorise what you should think about when a disclosure starts to be given.

Checklist: What to do when receiving a disclosure

The trainer needs to think about the following:

- Is it appropriate for the disclosure to take place in the group?
- It may have to be stopped if other members of the group become distressed.
- Does the disclosee need some space after the disclosure?
- Should the group have a time out after the disclosure has taken place?
- The need to spend time with the disclosee.
- How best to support the disclosee.
- Does the disclosee need future help/support/advice?
- Who is the best person to give this support?
- Are there any implications for the disclosee or for the work situation?
- Does information need to be shared?

Ongoing support can be important for participants who disclose on a course. It is very easy for a trainer to feel that s/he should be the person because s/he has received the disclosure. This can create problems as support may be needed regularly and for a lengthy period of time, and the trainer will probably not have the capacity to take on this role. So who could offer support? The following list offers some suggestions:

SUPPORT FOR PEOPLE WHO HAVE DISCLOSED

- Training officer

- Line manager

- Counsellor within the organisation

- Independent counsellor

- Independent therapist

- Support groups for survivors of abuse

- Specialist organisations

The trainer should be familiar with national and local organisations and groups which can offer specialist help. Participants may need help in regard to current/previous child abuse, domestic violence, sexual violence, harassment, bullying.

Picking up on abuse or bad practice

A trainer can pick up on the fact that abuse or bad practice is occurring within the organisation. This can happen in several ways:

- After going through definitions and categories of abuse, a participant can suddenly realise that a certain action/behaviour they have been engaging in is abusive. It is when people start to think about and discuss the more subtle forms of abuse that they become concerned about themselves or colleagues. Here are some examples:

    Three care staff from a supported accommodation project working with adults with learning disabilities said they would definitely not use nicknames anymore until they had checked it out with the service users.

> Staff working in a day centre had been told by the manager that a 'rule' which had to be observed was that service users whilst in the centre were not allowed to drink from a pop bottle or can.

> People with mental health problems were told they could not watch television in the mornings.

> In a nursing home, care staff had accepted the matron's rules of padlocking the fridges and freezer at night and not allowing residents food or drink after 7.00p.m.

- Participants talk about what they are doing and refuse to accept that their practices are bad. This can happen when someone has worked for a long period of time (e.g. care assistant working in the same home for the past 20 years) and has previously refused to come on any training courses, so has not developed different ways of working over the years. Examples:

> Care assistant working with residents who are demented says: 'you have to treat them like children'.

> 'When they're asleep we always go into their rooms and put our hands under their bums to see if they're wet. We wake them up if they need changing'.

> 'Can't see the point of care plans. We've never had them in our place. We know how to do care'.

- Through discussions it may become apparent that mangers are not doing their jobs properly or are in fact abusing staff. A problem area is that the trainer can be teaching participants about good practice, policy and procedures, but their managers might not have undertaken the same training and are therefore adopting different approaches. Examples:

> Manager is not convening case conferences after abuse investigations. He has what he calls 'group gatherings' to discuss future monitoring.

> Manager is bullying social worker and telling her 'all your work is rubbish'.

> Manager tells staff working with younger adults with challenging behaviour 'It's part of your job to be hit and sworn at. If you don't like it, go and work in Woolies.'

- Participants may talk about their own values or hold viewpoints which give the trainer cause for concern. Ground rule 4 (Chapter 4) states that participants will respect each other's views and not criticise, but there will be times when the trainer will have concerns about a participant and perhaps question how these values/views affect work practices. Sometimes, it is more constructive to discuss this with the individual outside of the group; otherwise s/he may see it as being criticised or humiliated in front of the group. Examples are where a participant believes that:

> 'Rape is about sexual gratification; power and control doesn't come into it.'

> 'A young person would not have sex with a pensioner because they're not attractive enough. It's not a turn on.'

> 'Old people shouldn't be allowed to have sex. It's nasty.'

> 'If they have learning difficulties, then their parents should manage their money 'cos they're not right in the head are they?'

> 'A slap never hurt anyone. A good pasting never did me any harm.'

It is important for the trainer to be clear about what his/her concerns are if this is going to be reported. The trainer has to be honest. If s/he has concerns these must be discussed with the individual or the group as a whole if appropriate. If the trainer is going to break confidentiality, then this must be discussed before the end of the course.

The trainer's options are – as previously when handling a disclosure – to report to the training officer or line manager. However, sometimes other actions will be needed; that is, the matter will be taken higher or elsewhere. Consequently, other people/organisations may become involved, e.g.

- senior managers within the organisation
- UKCC (United Kingdom Central Council) for Nursing, Midwifery and Health Visiting
- Registration and Inspection Unit
- harassment officers
- trade union representative.

If difficulties do arise on a course, it is advisable for the trainer to write notes about what happened during or immediately after the course whilst the incidents/comments are fresh in the mind. This is because the trainer may be asked for a full written report at a later date. If you run training courses throughout a working week it can be difficult to recall precise comments, times of incidents etc weeks later. Basically, it is about keeping accurate written records about what has happened.

TRAINER TIPS

- Always carry a notebook which can be used to record problems/difficulties on a course.

- Write incidents/comments up at break times if you have concerns.

- Write proper notes after the course has finished.

Unacceptable behaviour on a course

Participants can behave badly on a course for all sorts of reasons:

- They do not want to be there.

- They have been told they *have* to do the course.

- They are feeling uncomfortable about having to talk about abuse.

- They have personal experience of abuse.

- They do not like having to think about their own work practices.

- They have something to hide.

- They have problems with the trainer (maybe because of style of training, age, gender, race).

The trainer should try not to take this personally, but ask a fundamental question: 'What is making this person behave like this?'

It is hard when someone is making your job very difficult to remain calm and rational, but is necessary to take steps to find out the root cause of this behaviour. A participant can make life hell for a trainer by:

- being overtly rude/verbally aggressive

- constantly sighing, yawning, fidgeting

- looking bored/disinterested/fed up

- talking loudly to other members of the group whilst the trainer is presenting information

- challenging absolutely *everything* the trainer says

- denying that abuse exists

- repeatedly refusing to participate in exercises/discussions without giving a valid reason

- doing other work/tasks during the course (e.g. writing a work report which was 'more important than listening to this'; doing a crossword in the newspaper).

The trainer has to make the decision whether to confront the behaviour in the group or take the participant to one side. When I have challenged (in a constructive way) the person in the group, I can say that on most occasions s/he has behaved after that. Where it has been obvious that a person resents having to attend the course and bad behaviour persists, I have asked them to leave. I am glad to say that no one has ever done that.

Bad behaviour can be directed not towards the trainer but to other participants. This does need to be challenged in the group. I have only ever had one occasion when I had to stop the course because of what one participant was doing and saying to the rest of the group. The course was stopped for an hour whilst myself and a manager dealt with the abusive participant, who was immediately suspended. Time then had to be taken to talk to the other members of the group individually (luckily it was a small group of eight people), some of whom were very distraught and upset. I then ran a group discussion about what had happened and to ascertain whether it was appropriate to continue with the rest of the course, because all the participants were in a very emotional state. They chose to carry on. A lot of support work had to be undertaken in the following weeks with the participants when they were back in their workplaces.

I must emphasise that this has been worst experience ever and it is very unlikely that a trainer will have such an encounter. The lesson from this is that you have to do what you think is right at the time. You need to be able to think and act quickly.

TRAINER TIP

- If you find yourself in a quandary and need time to think, give the group a time-out (Ground rule 5).

After the event

If a trainer does have a hard time because difficult issues arise during a course, it is very necessary for him/her to talk it through with a designated support person (see Chapter 3). For inexperienced trainers this will be part of their professional development. So, when pools of trainers meet to review, time should be allocated on the agenda to discuss the problems which have arisen. Each trainer should gain support from other members of the pool as well as the leader. Experienced trainers can also face problems and they also need to talk to someone about what has happened; hence the reason to have an established support system for debriefing.

References

Pritchard, J. (2000) *The Needs of Older Women: Services for Victims of Elder Abuse and Other Abuse.* Bristol: Policy Press.

Pritchard, J. (1996) *Working with Elder Abuse: A Training Manual for Home Care, Residential and day Care Staff.* London: Jessica Kingsley Publishers.

Chapter 7

Problems for the Trainer

There are going to be many different types of trainer to be found in every pool; that is, they will all come with different levels of experience. Although I said earlier that I think it is preferable to have some experience in working with adult abuse, I know the reality is that there will be workers who put themselves forward for the pool who have never worked with adult abuse. Consequently, each individual trainer will face different kinds of problems when developing their skills as a trainer in adult abuse work. In this chapter I wish to discuss some of the most common problems I see trainers encounter as they train and then provide training courses on adult abuse.

Inexperience

Many people who volunteer to become a trainer have never had any experience of providing training and openly admit they are terrified of standing up in front of a group of people. Why do they put themselves through all this you may well ask? Probably because they think they have something to offer and it is something they want to do. So those are both very positive reasons for becoming a trainer.

When potential trainers admit their fears it is important to spend time discovering in what situations they have previously presented information to groups of people and then to build on these experiences. For example, people will have had to present in:

- work-related meetings, e.g. team meetings, case reviews, case conferences, ward rounds

- college seminars

- training sessions where they have been participants
- union meetings.

It can be helpful to ask participants to think of situations where they have had to present information to a group of people in a setting, which is not work-related. They might find this hard at first but eventually will think of examples and will see they have skills that could be used in training. Some examples I have been given are:

- presenting the costs of coach hire to a group of mothers at a crèche, who are organising a day trip to the sea-side
- presenting a Treasurer's report to the AGM at the local tennis club
- discussing a book at a reading group.

Exercise 7.1 on page 121 can be used to help participants realise how they have presented information in a group and to build their confidence.

When training trainers it is crucial to spend time letting people vent their worst fears and anxieties, but then to constructively build their confidence. One way to do this is for them to rehearse and use role-play situations.

Fear

We all fear things. Some common fears of people who have not trained before are:

- 'I won't keep their attention.'
- 'They'll be bored.'
- 'My mind will go blank.'
- 'I won't be able to answer their questions.'
- 'I won't be able to get it all in to the time.'
- 'I'll get through it too quickly and have time left over.'
- 'I dread having to handle disclosure.'
- 'What if I have to deal with a really difficult person?'

Potential trainers want reassurance and consequently it is very necessary to take them through practical ways of dealing with these situations. It is no use saying 'You'll be fine', 'You'll deal with it as it arises', etc. It is better to anticipate situations and develop strategies to cope with them. Exercise 7.2 may be used to achieve this (p.122).

BUILDING ON EXISTING SKILLS

Objective

To build confidence in presentation skills by reflecting back on situations where information has been relayed to a group of people.

Participants

Split participants into small groups c4–5.

Time

25 minutes in small groups; 30 minutes for feedback in large group.

Equipment

Flipchart paper and pens.

Task

Participants are asked to think about situations both in their personal and working lives where they have had to present information to a group of people. They should:

- make a list of the types of meeting

- describe what was good about the experience

- describe what was bad about the experience

- make a list of skills which were utilised during that meeting.

Feedback

Discussion in large group. Leader to collate the lists of skills and relate them to training skills.

ALLAYING FEARS

Objective

For trainers to confront their worst fears about what could happen during a training course.

Participants

Exercise to be done in pairs for stage 1. Then groups of four for stage 2.

Time

Timings will depend on how many people are involved in the pool. The role-plays may take a long time, so that this exercise might last a half day.

Equipment

Flipchart paper and pens

Task

Stage 1

Participants are asked to think about the situations they fear and would have difficulty in handling. They discuss this in pairs and list the fears on the flipchart sheet. After 10 minutes pairs are asked to join up into groups of four.

Stage 2

The two pairs compare their lists and then work on each fear. On a separate sheet of flipchart paper, stategies are developed to cope with the situations.

Stage 3

Role play within the large group. Each member of the group will have the opportunity to be the trainer. Other members of the group will act out some difficult behaviours that have been presented by the work done in pairs.

Feedback

Discussion in large group about the role-plays, i.e. what worked well and what did not. Leader to collate the list of strategies, which can be typed up and distributed to the pool members for future reference.

Lack of confidence

Some workers will have had experience of training and will not be as nervous as their colleagues; some may even feel slightly confident because 'I have done this before'. I think it is good to have some nervousness. No matter how experienced and knowledgeable you are, you need to have the adrenalin pumping in order to make you perform well. Trainers are dangerous if they become overly confident or too complacent. Training is like acting; you are performing for an audience and this is why trainers feel physically and emotionally drained at the end of the day. It is not an 'easy' job as some people seem to think.

Building confidence does not happen over night; it takes time. It is helpful to plan some training sessions close together, so that the sessions can be reflected upon and

---

TRAINER TIPS

To build confidence:

- Learn your material.

- Use aids, e.g. cards or notes, which can be used whilst delivering the training.

- Rehearse as much as possible:

    (i)   by yourself, e.g. in front of a mirror and with a tape recorder, so you can see and hear yourself

    (ii)   with your co-trainer

    (iii) in front of people, e.g. colleagues in the pool, who can give constructive criticism; other people you feel safe with, e.g. team members; family.

- Think about the comments which have been made and look at them positively not negatively.

- Consider the comments from evaluation forms and keep a record of them. Review them regularly and assess how you have progressed.

- After each course, make a list of:

    (i)   what you think you did really well

    (ii)   mistakes you made

    (iii) things you need to improve on.

Date each list made. Keep them and review them regularly.

---

analysed with the help of the leader who is training the trainers. Confidence will not be built effectively if there are massive time gaps, e.g. months between courses. Some useful tips are given on page 123.

Knowing the subject

In the list of tips, I have said that it is important to know the subject area. It is absolutely crucial that time is spent learning about the subject and the material that is to be presented. This learning process will take time; it cannot be crammed. As one becomes more familiar with materials, then confidence will build. The trainer needs to:

- read around subject of adult abuse, i.e. the theory
- be familiar with local policy and guidance
- be aware of current debates, practice issues
- keep up to date with national developments.

A suggested reading list is given in the Appendix, but to keep up to date trainers need to regularly do literature searches and read journals, magazines and newsletters of relevant organisations. I know people will moan about the fact that again this will take up more time, but it is necessary in order to be an effective trainer.

Not knowing

One of the greatest fears for a trainer is that you are going to be made to look stupid because you do not know something. I am always emphasising to people that one person cannot know everything. I am supposed to be 'the expert on abuse', but I am the first to admit there are many things I struggle with and sometimes I just do not know what the answer is. I do not think there is anything wrong in admitting:

- you do not know something
- you cannot answer a question
- you are unsure.

If you can find out in the future, then say that and do it! It is much better to admit openly that you do not know something rather than waffle on and try to cover up. If you do, then you lose your credibility. It is better to be honest; participants will have more respect for you. With adult abuse work there are so many dilemmas, that sometimes there is no right answer. Workers sometimes come on a course expecting the trainer to give them all the right answers and to resolve issues they have been struggling with. Adult abuse is an extremely complex issue; there are no simple answers and sometimes situations will remain unresolved.

Presentation skills

Everybody has different styles of presentation and for someone new to training, it is important to experiment. You need to feel comfortable with the style you adopt. There are many things to think about:

- Format for presentation.

- Do you feel more comfortable sitting or standing?

- Choice of equipment/aids. Are you going to use OHPs or flipchart as you speak? Will you need notes?

- Body language. How will you stand? Remember to fight bad habits (e.g using hands too much, walking around in circles, rocking motions).

- Voice. Speak loudly enough, clearly, slightly slower than normal, using intonation and emphases.

- Eye contact. It is imperative to engage with every member of the group. Do not focus on one spot in the room.

Keeping attention

It is important to keep people's attention during a training course, but in some ways it is even more difficult for the adult abuse trainer because some participants might deliberately 'turn off', perhaps because they feel uncomfortable.

Many workers who attend courses find it hard to sit in one place for hours on end. This is because usually they are being very active at work, running from one task to another (e.g. home care assistant, care worker, district nurse, ward nurse). So it is crucial that participants are 'kept moving'. If it is a full day, then it is good to use a mix of training methods; that is, presentations intermingled with group work, case studies, videos, role plays (See Chapter 5). It is important to keep the group work focused. Participants hate it when trainers say 'I want you to break into groups and talk about...'. Specific tasks need to be set.

TRAINER TIPS

- Use a variety of methods.

- Do not make each session too long.

- Have frequent short breaks.

- Afternoons need to be activity-based.

We all know about the 'graveyard' period after lunch – the trainer's nightmare. It is really important to keep the afternoon activity-based. Do not give long presentations if at all possible (although occasionally constraints on time make this impossible) and avoid showing videos straight after lunch. The same rules apply at the end of the afternoon. People might perk up mid-afternoon, but you lose them again at the end of the day, when they will be tired and emotionally drained. It is good to have a small group exercise during the last session so that people have to actively think; if they are sitting in a large group for a plenary session people will opt out because they are tired.

Time management

New trainers dread not being able to gauge time. Constant fears might be:

- Have I got enough material?

- Can I speak for long enough?

- What if I cannot control someone/group and they talk too much?

It is very important for a trainer to keep watching the time, but without making it obvious to the group. It is helpful to wear a watch that has a large face, i.e. you can see the hands clearly from a fair distance. Also, it is good to have a clock on the wall in the training room. From time to time you will have to work in a room where there is no clock at all, so I always carry a medium-sized alarm clock in my training bag that I can place somewhere in my line of vision.

When planning sessions for a training course, it is always good to allow extra time in case discussion does flow well. It is helpful to carry extra materials so that if you have an unresponsive group, you can put in an additional exercise to try to get them going.

It is better to be honest at the outset of the course and say that you will allow time for discussion and will aim to go at the group's pace, but acknowledge that there is a certain amount of material you must get through and there may be occasions when you will have to terminate the discussion in order to complete the training. This is more likely to occur in half-day sessions, when time is very tight. During the course of a full day, you have more flexibility and can adapt by shortening breaks/lunch hours, having a time-out to compensate. Pacing the course will come with experience and as you grow more confident, you will feel easier about moving people on. It has to be done in a sensitive manner and politely – not abruptly – and it is helpful to reiterate why you are having to do this.

Problem people

The trainer can never predict what is going to face them on the day. Every group of participants is different. It is important to remember that it takes time to get to know a group and how it presents in the first hour may be very different from how it presents later in the day. Participants have to get to know the trainer and each other, and build their own trust and confidence. Participants might be coming with their own 'baggage' – for example they may feel:

- dread about the subject of the course

- out of their depth (especially when you have a mix of staff, e.g. residential and home care staff on multi-disciplinary training with managers, social workers, community psychiatric nurses, police etc)

- fears about having to work in a group with strangers

- inadequate because they have difficulty with reading or writing.

Basically, it takes time for a group to gell, and the first hour or so can make an inexperienced trainer feel uncomfortable, because the group may be quiet and unresponsive. The trainer must remember that it is a testing-out time for them too. Hence the reason for trying to get the group talking early on (but my preference is *not* for what I call 'silly' exercises to introduce themselves; it is better to use exercises that have a purpose related to learning about abuse and which will engage participants so that they meet each other whilst learning too).

The problem people who the trainer may face are those who:

- dominate

- talk too much

- challenge everything the trainer says in a very negative way

- present aggressively

- do not engage at all.

For someone who is overtly a problem for the trainer and the group, it is best to challenge that person in the group. If the problems persist, then the trainer needs to speak to the person outside the group. Exercise 7.3 will help trainers develop ways of challenging people in a constructive way.

In some organisations morale is extremely low and workers can use the training course to vent their feelings to the trainer because they feel that no one else listens to them. They can also enjoy the opportunity to talk to colleagues who are also fed up with the workload, organisation etc. I think it is fine for workers to offload, but again the trainer has to time-limit this. The trainer has to acknowledge the conditions and circumstances that are affecting workers, but must not get sucked into it. I am frequently told by workers who are fed up that it is fine for me to talk about good practice but because of the way the organisation expects the workers to function it is not possible to implement what I am suggesting; mainly because of lack of time, staff, budgets and so on. I do believe very strongly that workers have to take some responsibility for themselves. It is all too easy to blame the organisation or other people within it.

Development and evaluation

In Chapters 6 and 7 I have raised a lot of issues and problems that could face a trainer and I have also made suggestions about how to address these difficulties. It is vital that the trainer's performance is evaluated (which will be discussed in the following chapter), but the trainer must also evaluate him/herself on a regular basis. The leader who is training the trainers should provide sessions where reflection on performance can take place. Any trainer, whether experienced or inexperienced, needs to constantly review their performance and improve their weaker skills. This can only be done with constructive criticism and good ongoing support.

CHALLENGING DIFFICULT PEOPLE

Objective

To develop ways of confronting a person who is disrupting the group/training session.

Participants

Split participants into small groups of about 4–5.

Time

15 minutes to work in groups.

Equipment

The trainer needs to have prepared some scenarios in advance.

Each group is given two scenarios.

Flipchart paper and pens.

Task

Each group is given two scenarios where a person is presenting a problem on a course. The group is asked to make a list of actual sentences which could be used to address the problem.

Feedback

Each group feeds back to the large group. People are asked to comment if they do not like any of the sentences or to add to the suggestions.

Chapter 8

Evaluation

When an organisation is providing training on adult abuse, a vital part of the process is to undertake proper and thorough evaluation of the:

- training programme that has been developed

- individual training courses which are provided

- trainer(s) who are providing the courses.

Organisations cannot sit back and think the job has been done once a training programme is up and running. The lead person needs to develop an evaluation system that is going to find out exactly:

- what has been provided, i.e. course content

- whether the original programme met the set objectives

- whether it has been cost effective

- how the trainers have performed

- what the training needs of the workforce are for the future.

The training programme

The organisation will have developed aims and objectives in regard to what they wanted to achieve through training (see Chapter 1), and an evaluation of the programme should produce evidence of whether these original targets have been met (see 'Learning Outcomes' on p.27, and Example 2 on p.134). In many organisations there will be a working party or sub-group formed, whose remit will be to work on adult abuse training. Such groups should meet regularly to review what has taken place. Therefore, the lead person for training needs to take a systematic approach to evaluation and be able to feedback to the group. Training programmes should not be static; they need to be reviewed regularly and a full evaluation needs to be undertaken annually.

To begin the process of evaluation the lead person should undertake a training-needs analysis. The organisation has to make it clear to managers that training in general is important. Good practice should ensure that the training needs of staff are fed back systematically to the training section so that appropriate training courses can be provided. Education is one of the main functions of supervision; managers should be promoting professional development through education and training. There should be no reason at all why training profiles cannot be developed during supervision sessions.

A training-needs analysis should be developed specifically for the adult abuse programme (but I know this is often not done in depth). At the same time the lead person should be developing evaluation systems that are to be implemented once the training courses begin.

Evaluation of courses

Courses need to be evaluated both for the purposes of the trainer and for the organisation. Any good trainer will want to know if the structure and content have met the needs of the participants and the organisation and whether anything needs to be changed in the future. The organisation needs to know whether the right sort of course is being provided, i.e. are participants being equipped to do the job?; are they competent?

Evaluations can be done verbally or in written form. Most trainers will take some verbal feedback at the end of a course, but one never knows how honest participants are going to be and an added factor is that by the end of the day participants are often tired and just want to go home. Consequently, written evaluations can be rushed 'just to get it done with'. It is important that the trainer allows enough time at the end of a course for verbal feedback (and to check out if people are feeling OK – see Chapter 4) and written evaluations. It is important for the trainer to stress the value of evaluation;

many participants have no idea why they are required to engage in this activity or what happens to the evaluation forms!

Over the years I have used numerous evaluations forms designed by organisations. I cannot say I have been really happy with them, because there is always 'something else' I want to know. The way evaluation forms are structured often 'leads' the participant; people rarely fill in the 'Other comments' section. The standard evaluation form includes questions in order to obtain comments regarding:

- pre-course information

- venue

- catering

- parking facilities

- course objectives and learning outcomes (e.g.were they met?)

- expectations of the participant (e.g.were they met?)

- relevance to job

- trainer (style, presentation, methods, aids, ability to communicate)

- anti-discriminatory practice.

Organisations have different ways of evaluating on forms. Some will use open questions only:

- 'Which aspect of the course did you find most helpful?'

- 'Which aspect of the course not helpful?'

- 'Are there any changes that you could suggest that might improve or develop this particular course further?'

Others use scales to grade responses.

EXAMPLE I

How satisfied were you with the following aspects of the Training Course you have attended? Please give a Satisfaction Rating in the right hand box using the scale below

ISSUE   RATING

- The course content was relevant to your learning needs. ☐

- Course objectives were clearly stated and easily understood. ☐

- Course objectives were achieved. ☐

- The course encouraged you to contribute using your previous knowledge and experience. ☐

- Attention was paid to anti-discriminatory practice and use of non-discriminatory language. ☐

- Positive attitudes towards learning were encouraged by the trainer. ☐

- The material was presented in such a way as to be clear and easily understood. ☐

- The style of the presenter was appropriate. ☐

- Effective use was made of training resources e.g. flipchart, video etc. ☐

Totally dissatisfied	*Not very satisfied*	*Quite satisfied/ satisfied*	*Very satisfied*
1	*2*	*3*	*4*

✔

EXAMPLE 2

Did the course achieve the learning outcomes?

Learning Outcome	Poor	Fair	Good	Very good	Excellent
1. Raised awareness					
2. Developed skills					
3. Examined values and attitudes					
4. Gained overview of legislation					
5. Gained good working knowledge					
6. Achieved clear understanding of local policy and procedure					

EXAMPLE 3

1. How did you find the level of the course?

Too basic ☐   About right ☐   Too advanced ☐

2. What was the standard of the trainer?

Poor ☐   Fair ☐   Good ☐   Very good ☐   Excellent ☐

Or there will be a mix of both, i.e. scales followed by questions:

EXAMPLE 4

Looking at the course objectives how were they met?

Well ☐   Quite well ☐   Not well ☐   Poorly ☐

If you felt any objectives were not met adequately please comment below:

EXAMPLE 5

Standard of trainer's presentation:

Very poor	Poor	Average	Good	Very good
1	2	3	4	5

Comment on:

   (a)   The overall standard of the material and information that was given to you

   (b)   Skills and methods used by the trainer

If questions are to be used, they have to be designed carefully so that the course participant is going to give the sort of information required. If the questions are too broad or unfocused the evaluations may be meaningless. The participant needs to understand the value and purpose of the evaluation. Some of the general questions illustrated above are too general, which from a trainer's point of view is not going to be helpful.

A method I have developed over the years is to get participants to write a letter to me. I ask them to write their own evaluation of the course based upon whatever is going through their minds at the time. By this 'free-style' approach I find I get a more reflective and true account from people. This method is particularly useful for the trainer and his/her self assessment. This is because participants are not being led to think in a certain way but also they have to really think before writing. The trainer can prepare sheets beforehand or ask the participants to get a blank piece of paper and put at the top details of the course attended (see page 137).

The trainer should stress that the letter can be signed or remain anonymous. It is helpful for the trainer to explain why s/he values the evaluations and what actually happens to the sheets; participants do not feel they are wasting their time if they know the forms are going to be taken seriously. Using the letter method I have found that often participants will write a lot more than they would normally. If the organisation has a standard evaluation form, the letter-type evaluation can be done in addition so as to meet the requirements of the organisation and the trainer.

Ongoing evaluation

One evaluation form completed at the end of the day is not sufficient to evaluate a course properly. The evaluation process needs to be more thorough and systematic. Some years ago as an independent consultant, I organised training courses for voluntary organisations that worked with clients from the local probation service in a specified geographical area. My remit was to identify training needs, organise courses and evaluate both courses and trainers. So I have had the experience of managing and organising training as well as providing it. One thing I developed during that piece of work was an ongoing evaluation system, which I think could be adopted by any organisation that is providing adult abuse training for its workers. Different evaluation forms were designed for dissemination at various stages as shown below. In addition a set number of telephone interviews were conducted, both with participants and their line managers, who were selected at random.

136

EXAMPLE EVALUATION LETTER

Date:

Title of course:

Dear *(Trainer's name)*

SYSTEM OF EVALUATION

Stage 1 – end of course

Evaluation form 1 – completed by all participants on a course.

Stage 2 – one month after the course was completed

Evaluation form 2 – sent out to all participants.
Telephone interviews with a selected number of participants.

Stage 3 – three months after the course was completed

Evaluation form 3a – sent out to a selected number of participants who agreed to participate in the evaluation exercise.

Evaluation form 3b – sent out to line managers of the participants who were selected to complete form 3a.

Telephone interviews with a selected number of participants, who were not completing written evaluations.

Stage 4 – six months after the course was completed

Forms 3a and 3b – sent out again to the same participants and line managers.
Telephone interviews with other participants

Evaluation forms 1 and 2 included questions to get views on:

- pre-course information (original flyer, objectives and learning outcomes, programme, venue, directions)
- location of venue; training room; catering
- objectives and learning outcomes
- course content
- trainer
- materials provided
- integration of equal opportunities
- application of learning on the course to job/work
- future training needs
- current training programme.

EVALUATION FORM – EXAMPLE QUESTIONS

- Was the knowledge gained from the course useful?

  Yes ☐   No ☐

If yes, in what way?

- Was the information you received relevant to your work?

  Yes ☐   No ☐

- Did you share any of the information you received on the course with your:

Manager ☐   Colleagues ☐   Users ☐   Others (please specify) ☐

- Have your behaviour/work practices with any of the above mentioned people changed in any way as a result of the course:

  Yes ☐   No ☐

If yes, in what way?

- Have you put what you learnt from the course into practice at work?

  Yes ☐   No ☐

If yes, can you give some examples of how you have done this (related either to knowledge gained or skills learnt):

© Jacki Pritchard 2001

- Have you used any of the materials you received from the course?

    Yes ☐   No ☐

Which materials?

How have you used them?

- Has your practice changed in any way as a result of the course?

    Yes ☐   No ☐

If yes, in what way?
(Give specific examples if you can)

- Have you done anything better or more effectively as a result of the course?

    Yes ☐   No ☐

Please explain how you have done this.

- Do you think the training received on this course has made a difference to the service you are providing to users?

  Yes ☐   No ☐

In what way?

- Looking back, would you say now that there were any gaps in the course?

  Yes ☐   No ☐

What are they?

- Are there any specific topics/issues/subjects areas that should have been included in the course?

  Yes ☐   No ☐

Please specify:

- Will you be using any knowledge/information gained from the course in your future work/practice?

  Yes ☐   No ☐

How will you do this?

Evaluation form 3a asked participants to reflect on the course before answering detailed questions. The evaluation began by asking about the level of the course and the standard of the trainer. This was important because responses often changed with time after the participant had reflected on what they had learnt. The rest of the evaluation form asked questions about the course content and how the knowledge gained had been implemented back at the workplace. In using this type of evaluation form, questions need to be very focused and participants must be asked to give examples to illustrate exactly what they mean.

Examples

When designing questions for evaluating adult abuse courses, more specific questions could be designed about actual work practices; that is, as a result of the course, how are participants currently dealing with:

- referrals
- investigations
- liaising with other professionals, agencies
- obtaining specific information (e.g. legal matters, assessments)
- case conferences
- development of protection plans
- monitoring and reviewing systems.

It is also useful to know when information became useful for the participants; that is:

- Were there certain elements of the course that were implemented immediately once back at work?
- Were there certain elements of the course that were implemented at a later date?

Developing this system does take a lot of time and hard work. A great deal of thought needs to go into the questions that are going to be used on the evaluation forms in order to obtain the right sort of information, which can then be used for proper analysis.

Evaluation form 3b was developed for line managers and asked them to consider whether the worker's practices had changed in any way as a direct result of the training course. Both 3a and 3b were then sent out six months after the course, and it was evident that respondents' answers did change with time.

When evaluating the usefulness of basic raising-awareness courses concerned with adult abuse, there is a need to know whether workers are able to:

- understand what is meant by abuse

- recognise abuse

- follow the required procedures.

Sometimes it is only when participants are back at work that they realise what:

- was missing on a course

- they need to improve in or have more knowledge about

- they have not understood when trying to put policy into practice.

Also, their managers and colleagues should notice if their practices have changed. Therefore, opinions have to be sought from managers as well as ensuring that training issues are linked into the supervision and appraisal processes.

It is helpful for the lead person and trainer to know:

- issues/dilemmas that people struggle with back at the workplace

- what a course needs to address in more detail

- what subject areas/information were difficult to assimilate/retain.

The Trainer's evaluation

It is also important that the organisation obtains an evaluation of a course from the trainer's point of view. I am often asked to complete a trainer's evaluation form regarding the form in regard to:

- information provided before the course, e.g. about venue, participants

- administrative matters

- venue/catering

- the delivery of the course

- the participants

- problems

- improvements/changes to the course for the future

- the size of group – was it appropriate?

- the need for follow-on/related courses.

The trainer

It is important for a trainer to continually evaluate his/her own performance and professional development. The trainer needs to know from the participants' point of view how s/he has performed during a course. Also the trainer will have had his/her own objectives and ways of delivering the necessary information. Participants have different styles of learning and the style of the trainer may not have suited the needs of some participants. The trainer has to think on his/her feet during a course; it is usually possible to tell when something is not sinking in or not making sense to someone. The trainer has to check this out at regular intervals through the course. I use phases like 'Does that make sense?'; 'Am I making sense?'; 'Are you clear about the procedure?'; 'Do you need to me to go over anything again?'; 'Are there any questions?' When participants are finding it difficult, the trainer has to adapt and use different methods of training.

All trainers need to be observed regularly as part of the evaluation process. Trainers can gain a good reputation but anyone employing that person or buying them in (as for independent trainers) needs to see what they are actually doing. I have been involved in evaluating performances of trainers and on occasions have found 'the experts' have not in fact been very good or have not been doing what they were supposed to do (i.e. course content was very different to what was wanted by the organisation). It can be like the 'emperor's new clothes' syndrome, i.e. people are afraid to say what they really see – especially if that person has a good reputation and is seen as important.

As an independent trainer, I like a training officer to participate in my courses to see what I actually do. I also like to co-train because your colleague can give you feedback. Feedback from another trainer is always invaluable.

There is the danger that if a trainer is repeating a course very regularly, s/he could become bored, complacent or stale. This is another reason why I believe that trainers should not train more than three days a week – especially on the same subject.

As a pool of trainers is being developed it is important that each trainer is monitored. It is helpful for them to be shadowed initially, but then after delivering courses on their own for about six months they need an expert evaluation. This should to be done by someone independent, not someone they know. The trainer will be watched and evaluated by the independent evaluator. Written evaluations from other courses will also be used and any other evidence that the evaluator thinks necessary. The evaluation will then be written in the form of a report and presented to the trainer and the person responsible for the pool of trainers. Objectives can be set to improve performance.

Self evaluation is important. The leader of the pool may incorporate Exercise 9.1 (p.146) in one of the support sessions for trainers. It can be a follow-on exercise from the original Tree Exercise (Chapter 3 – Exercise 3.1.) or it can be undertaken as an independent exercise itself.

Some practitioners realise early on that training is not for them – some drop out during the training-the-trainers courses; others give up during the first six months. Some will be bad trainers, but think they are good. When this happens, honesty must prevail and work needs to be done to counsel them out of doing any further training. Other trainers may have faults or weaknesses, which can be worked on, but again the evaluator has to be honest about this and there needs to be an agreed plan of action.

Evaluating the pool

The trainers within a pool will be assessed individually but the organisation needs to evaluate the pool as a whole. The basic question to be asked is: 'Is the pool working?'

Annual evaluations should take place because it is very likely that circumstances will change. For example, within the first year of a pool, developing trainers may have dropped out. If the organisation has not developed an ongoing recruitment strategy, then further thought will have to be given to recruitment and training. Pools will function in different ways and a year on, the organisation may realise that they want the pool to be different in some way. Consequently, as with the evaluation of the training programme, the lead person will need to develop a system of evaluating the pool to find out whether it:

- has an adequate number of trainers (too few or too many?)
- is flexible enough, e.g. can it meet demand for training; do trainers mix and match etc.
- is well co-ordinated
- has sufficient training/resources/support for the trainers.

THE AUTUMN TREE EXERCISE

Objective

To help trainers in a pool to think how they have developed since starting to provide courses on adult abuse.

Participants

Participants will work by themselves initially.

Time

15 minutes to work by oneself; 15 minutes to present and discuss tree with rest of the group.

Equipment

Flipchart paper and pens.

Task

Participants are asked to draw a tree trunk on a flipchart sheet, with branches stemming from the right and left, but leaving the top of the tree bare. They are then asked to put leaves on the branches as follows:

- On the left-hand side – the skills and knowledge already possessed when joining the pool that could be useful in training on adult abuse. (Participants who did Exercise 3.1 and kept the tree can refer to the original drawing.)

- On the right-hand side – skills and knowledge developed since attending training-the-trainer sessions and providing courses on adult abuse.

At the top of the tree, participants are asked to identify:

- weaknesses

- skills they need to develop further

- gaps in knowledge

- things they are worried about.

Feedback

Participants are given time to present their trees to the rest of the group. The tree will be displayed on the flipchart stand. The Participants will talk about their tree, after which the rest of the group will comment.

© Jacki Pritchard 2001

Conclusion

Evaluation is not just about course participants filling in evaluation forms. The discussion above shows that the organisation providing training has to also develop thorough evaluation systems to ensure that the workforce continues to be trained and developed in order to work effectively with adult abuse. Good evaluation will ensure that training needs are identified and that effective trainers will provide courses to meet these needs. Some suggested reading on evaluation of training is given in the Appendix of this guide.

Chapter 9

Case Studies

This chapter includes a number of case studies that can be used in a variety of ways by a trainer whose time is limited or who has not had direct experience of working with abuse cases. They relate to different service user groups, all of whom are vulnerable adults. They can be used as they stand for basic discussion, or specific questions could be added in order to set tasks for small group work.

The trainer should adapt the material to suit the training needs of the participants, who will come from different backgrounds. Basically, they can be used to work on:

- types of abuse (categorisation)

- identification of abuse (signs and symptoms)

- procedures (what should be done).

Below I have listed some typical questions that could be used, depending on the objective of the exercise and the mix of participants. The trainer needs to pick out individual questions, not to use all of them for each exercise.

- Is this a case of abuse? If so, which category(ies) of abuse?

- Who should report this?

- Should an adult abuse investigation take place?

- What should happen next?

- What are the problem areas?

- What are the dilemmas?

- What would you do?

- Having read this case study, what thoughts are going through your mind?

- How do you think you would react if you had to deal with this situation?

- What would you struggle with?

- What more do you want to know?

- Are there any signs/indicators of abuse?

- Could they be signs/indicators of something else?

- If you were appointed investigating officer:

  (i)   What other information would you like to have access to or to gather yourself?

  (ii) What questions would you want to ask the alleged victim?

- Are any special assessments required?

- Should any action have been taken before this incident/situation was reached? If yes, what should have happened?

- What emotions are you feeling having read this case study?

Case Study I

Subject: Eleanor (age 24)

Eleanor has moderate learning disabilities; she can communicate very well and likes to be independent. She lives in supported accommodation and has been there for about six months.

About four months ago she started going to flower arranging classes every week at the local community centre. She seemed to really enjoy the classes at first and made a friend called Tricia. Tricia is older than Eleanor and lives locally with her husband, Paul, and two young children. Eleanor often goes to Tricia and Paul's house for tea.

Over the past month Eleanor has become moody. She seems very unhappy when she comes home from the classes but says she is 'all right'. She has also refused to go out with her other friends and now spends most of her time in her room.

Today her keyworker has put time aside to talk to Eleanor because both staff and service users are concerned about her. After some discussion Eleanor bursts into tears and says she is 'frightened of Tricia and Paul'. The worker probes further and eventually Eleanor says that Tricia and Paul have been taking money from her.

Case Study 2

Subject: Gregory (age 25)

Gregory has moderate learning disabilities and has lived in the current supported accommodation project, which is run by a voluntary organisation, for the past five years. Another man, Anthony, who is also in his mid 20s and also has moderate learning disabilities, has been living in the project for only three months.

It has been evident since they first met that Gregory and Anthony do not like each other. They often argue with each other in front of other services users and then do not talk to each other for days. The arguments seem to have got worse lately; both staff and other services users are getting pretty fed up. Staff who have known Gregory for a long time have commented how they have noticed changes in him; he is normally very passive and willing to get along with anybody. They say he has become argumentative and verbally and physically aggressive to staff and other service users.

Staff decide at a team meeting that the situation needs to be discussed both with Gregory and Anthony individually in the first instance. When the problem is discussed with Gregory he says he does not like Anthony because since being there he has always come into his bed at night and does 'naughty things'. No other information can be obtained from Gregory. Anthony has been asked about this and denies ever going into Gregory's room.

Case Study 3

Subject: Joshua (age 38)

Joshua is an Afro-Caribbean man who has severe learning disabilities and no verbal communication. He has lived in residential care ever since his family was killed in a car crash. An old friend of the family, Zachary, visits Joshua about two or three times a month.

Zachary has become extremely concerned about Joshua during the past six months because there have been so many changes in his behaviour and physical condition. Joshua, who is now always in bed whatever time of day Zachary visits, has started sucking his thumb and rocking in bed; on occasions he has been crying when Zachary has arrived on a visit. He does not seem to recognise Zachary any more, who describes him as being 'like a zombie now'. Zachary has also noticed that Joshua always smells of urine, his skin is 'very rough' and his hair is 'dry'. Zachary always brings creams and oils for Joshua and staff have been shown how to use these in the past.

When Zachary has voiced his concerns to staff, they say that 'Joshua is Joshua and you can't make him do anything he doesn't want to do'.

Case Study 4

Subject: Katie (aged 40)

Katie has severe learning disabilities and cannot communicate verbally. She has lived in supported accommodation since her mother died two years ago. Her only relative is her step-father, Mr Chambers.

Mr Chambers visits Katie once a week on a Sunday afternoon. He has an agreement, which was made with the social worker and not discussed with the project staff, that his taxi fares from home to the project will be paid for out of Katie's money and that any expenditure incurred on visits (e.g if they go out for a coffee, to the pictures, to eat etc) will also be paid for with Katie's money.

The workers in the project have discussed this and feel Katie is being financially abused. The social worker disagrees and says it is important that Katie has some contact with a family member. Mr Chambers has now started bringing his new partner to visit, so taxi fares and other costs have increased.

Case Study 5

Subject: Angela (aged 20)

In the past Angela has made allegations that she has been sexually abused by her father, uncle and brother. Nothing has ever been proven. She has had numerous social workers over the years and attended various day centres. She has never made any allegations about anyone else except her family. She currently lives in supported accommodation and attends a Social Education Centre. She occasionally has weekend stays with her family.

She returns home to the project house at 4.00 on a Friday afternoon and says that another service user has touched her breasts and put his hand in her knickers. She had told a worker at the Social Education Centre who responded by saying 'We all know about you and your storytelling'.

Angela is sobbing whilst talking about the incident once she is at home. She is very clear about the incident, where and when it happened. She says she does not want to return to the Social Education Centre ever again. A worker notices that Angela has broken fingernails and scratches on her hands.

Case Study 6

Subject: Monica (aged 47)

Monica has multiple sclerosis. She has been very ill during the past few weeks and is currently spending most of her time in bed. She lives with her husband, who is a police officer, and 17-year-old son who is studying for A levels at school. A social worker from the Physical Disability Team is involved and home care assistants currently go in twice a day to check on Monica whilst her husband and son are out.

The home care staff are very concerned about Monica. She cries a lot, which they put down to her 'being depressed about the MS', but they are more worried about the bruises and black eyes they are seeing frequently. Monica says that she frequently goes dizzy and falls when she gets out of bed to go to the toilet. They have reported this to the Home Care Manager but nothing seems to have been followed up.

Today when the home care assistants go in Monica has severe bruising and cuts on her face and a clump of hair is missing from her head. She says that her husband has attacked her. She goes on to say that this is not the first time but the attacks have gone on for years. Monica says she is 'petrified' of her husband, but does not want anything to be reported.

Case Study 7

Subject: Reg (aged 40)

Reg was left blind and severely disabled after a horrific car crash ten years ago. His wife left him two years ago, because she had 'had enough of being a carer' and wanted 'to have a life'. Reg is in receipt of a care package from social services and manages very well. He likes to have people visit him as much as possible. He has no family, but friends and neighbours pop in during the evenings. Reg says the days are very long when he is at home and not at the day centre. So his social worker has arranged for a volunteer, Frances, to visit once a week.

On recent visits the social worker has noticed that things have been missing in Reg's lounge – an antique vase, an oil painting on the wall, the stereo. Reg says that he has given these possessions to Frances because 'she is so kind and she has terrible problems at home'. Frances has been telling Reg that she is a single parent who is struggling to provide for her two children. Reg also discloses that he has been lending her money.

Case Study 8

Subject: Lisa Roberts (aged 19)

Lisa has cerebral palsy and continues to live with her family – mother, father, and two brothers, aged 13 and 15 years. A new social worker, Alice, has become involved with Lisa since she has started to injure herself on a regular basis. She has been cutting herself with various objects.

When the social worker visits, Mrs Roberts is unwilling to leave the room so Alice has never spoken to Lisa on her own. On her third visit Alice suggests that she takes Lisa out for a coffee in order to give her mother a break. Mrs Roberts reluctantly agrees.

As soon as Lisa gets in the car, she says she never wants to go back home. She discloses that her brothers continually make fun of her, her father hits her on occasions and her mother keeps her locked in her bedroom during the daytime. She admits that she has tried to kill herself.

Lisa's parents have a high profile in the local community. Her father is a local councillor and over the years her mother has done a lot of voluntary work at the local children's hospital and raised large amounts of money for children with cerebral palsy.

Case Study 9

Subject: Ben (aged 22)

Ben spent over a year in hospital receiving treatment for a head injury, which he sustained after falling when he was rock climbing. He has now returned home to live with his parents.

Whilst in the special head injury unit, Ben made good progress and he was a favourite of the nursing staff. His social worker, who visits once a week, has noticed a dramatic change in Ben. Since going home he has become very depressed and does not seem to want to make any effort. He refuses to do any of his exercises. The social worker is also concerned about his physical appearance; he is often in his pyjamas in the daytime and seems as though he is not being well cared for (he sometimes smells of urine, his fingernails are dirty, his hair is greasy).

His mother has given up her job as a teacher to care for Ben and she is obviously finding the change difficult to cope with. She talks openly to the social worker about resenting the fact she has had to give up her career and she does not like having to do the intimate physical tasks involved in caring for Ben. She feels very isolated because Ben's father works away a lot and there are no other family members living locally. She says friends also visit less frequently because 'they feel awkward'.

Case Study 10

Subject: Alan (aged 52)

From the age of 9, Alan suffered with severe leg ulcers; his condition worsened in adulthood and when he was 30 years old he had to have both legs amputated. Over the years he has worked occasionally, but has not worked at all for the past ten years. Nowadays he gets very depressed about his disability and has started to drink heavily. He spends most of his time in a wheelchair and refuses to transfer to a chair. He does not like people seeing him and is very rude to anyone who comes to the house. Consequently, neighbours and friends have stopped visiting. A social worker from the physical disability team visits once a month.

Margaret, Alan's wife, has a part-time job at the local fish and chip shop; she works lunchtimes 12.00 until 2.00. Alan resents Margaret leaving him alone, but Margaret feels desperate to get out of the house. Margaret has also started to drink; previously she had been tee-total. She now drinks as soon as she comes in during the afternoon and by the evening she is very drunk and incapable of cooking or helping Alan. When Alan has been drinking and is annoyed with Margaret he becomes verbally abusive to her. Margaret retaliates by hitting Alan either with her hand or with objects which are close by.

Alan and Margaret have one son, Jack, who lives abroad and has little contact with his parents.

This evening a neighbour has heard shouting and screaming and has called the police. When the police arrive they find Alan and Margaret unconscious; Alan is bleeding from a cut on his head.

Case Study 11

Subject: Harry (aged 49)

Harry has been known to the psychiatric services for several years. He was diagnosed as having Wernicke Korsakoff syndrome, which is an uncommon brain disorder almost always due to malnutrition that occurs in chronic alcohol dependence. Harry's memory is poor and he often becomes very anxious; he is extremely thin. He currently lives with his teenage son, Jason. His wife left the family home when Jason was a toddler; her whereabouts are unknown.

Several professionals have regular contact with Harry – social worker, community psychiatric nurse – and he is monitored via the local hospital.

They are all concerned by Harry's current state of health and the fact that he often presents as hungry and thirsty when visiting the hospital for appointments.

The police have now contacted the social worker because neighbours have repeatedly called the police out in the past two weeks, when they have heard shouting and furniture being thrown about. On the last occasion Harry admitted that Jason had tried to strangle him when he had refused to hand over money to go drinking. Harry refused to press charges against Jason.

Case Study 12

Subject: Donovan (aged 55)

Donovan has been diagnosed with aggravated depression; his history of depression goes back 18 years. The psychiatrist currently involved feels that everything has been done to help Donovan; all types of treatment have been administered over the years. He has attempted suicide on four occasions. He has not worked for the past five years.

Donovan lives with his wife, Elizabeth; they have no children. Donovan attends a day centre for people with mental health problems. He has told workers in the day centre that his wife regularly hits him. Today, an ambulance brings Donovan into the Accident and Emergency Department at the local hospital. On examination, the doctor finds that Donovan has different coloured bruises on the back of his neck, upper arms, lower back and buttocks. Elizabeth openly admits that she gave Donovan too much medication and that she hits him on a regular basis when she feels exasperated with him. She says she is 'the abused one' because he continually asks her to kill him.

Case Study 13

Subject: Martin (aged 25)

Martin uses a drop-in centre for people who have drug-related problems. He has developed a very good relationship with one of the workers, Jake. Martin and his girlfriend, Rachel, have been living on the streets for years; they are currently squatting in a derelict house.

Recently, Martin has been using the drop-in centre more frequently, which Rachel does not like. She is also a drug user but does not want to do anything about it, whereas Martin does want to stop. Recently, Martin has been able to tell Jake that he was sexually abused by both his father and mother when he was a small child and this was the reason for him leaving home at the age of 14.

When Martin comes to the drop-in centre today, he seems to be in a great deal of pain and the front of his jumper is saturated with blood. He admits to Jake that Rachel has slashed him with a knife; he has lacerations across his stomach. He goes on to say that Rachel has always been physically violent towards him since their relationship began.

Case Study 14

Subject: Julie (aged 32)

Julie has been known to the local social services departments for years. She has been diagnosed as schizophrenic. When she takes her medication she functions very well; she manages her bedsit and regularly attends a mental health day centre. When things are going well she usually stops taking her medication and admits she 'gets in a muddle'. The pattern is that she usually forms inappropriate relationships.

Last time she was sectioned, she met Luther on the hospital ward. Luther is a Schedule 1 offender and is said to have a personality disorder. When Julie went home, Luther moved into her bedsit. Julie returned to the day centre but her attendance was erratic. She presented with black eyes and bruises and never had any money on her to buy food or cigarettes. She then stopped coming to the day centre. Staff tried to visit her at home, but Luther would not let them in the door.

Neighbours have now told the social worker, who has also been refused entry, that they have often heard Julie screaming and the police have been called out on several occasions.

Case Study 15

Subject: Ali (21)

Ali is an Asian man who has mental health problems and currently resides in a halfway house with 5 other men, all of whom are white.

Ever since Ali came to live in the house, he has been the recipient of racist comments from people in the community (*not* from the other residents). At first he managed to ignore the comments, but gradually the situation has become worse.

There is now a gang of children aged between 9 and 11 years, who are continually tormenting him. They throw stones at the windows of the house, write graffiti on the front door, and have now started following Ali when he goes out in the morning to work at the local petrol station and in the evening when he comes home.

Ali has become very depressed. He started taking days off work but now refuses to go out at all. When a brick came through a window, another resident was cut by the broken glass. The police said nothing could be done because no one saw the cuplrit who threw the brick.

Case Study 16

Subject: Mrs Bryers (aged 68)

Mrs Bryers, who is agoraphobic, owns an old Victorian house which is divided into bedsits. Fred Lampton, aged 56, lives in one of these bedsits; he has not worked since he had an accident in a local factory six years ago. Mrs Bryers was slightly confused before she suffered a stroke and was admitted to hospital. Since the stroke she has been severely confused, but does recognise Fred and is always pleased to see him when he visits her every day in hospital.

Fred manages Mrs Bryers' finances and has done since he finished working. He is a signatory for her bank and building societies in which she has over £50,000. Before the hospital admission he cashed her pension, collected the rents from the other tenants, did the shopping and paid the bills.

Mrs Bryers is still in hospital recovering from the stroke when Fred announces that they are going to be married. He has bought Mrs Bryers an engagement ring with her own money. Nursing staff are convinced that Mrs Bryers does not really understand what is happening to her and that Fred is 'just after her money'. Mrs Bryers keeps saying she wants to go home.

165

Case Study 17

Subject: Lucinda (age 90)

Lucinda has started coming in for respite care every six weeks. She lives with one of her two sons, Edgar, who is in his 60s and says he is finding it hard to cope with his mother, who has 'always been difficult'.

Lucinda presents as slightly confused, but presents no behaviour problems until she goes to bed. She insists on having her walking stick in bed with her and screams if anyone enters the bedroom when she is still awake. One night she hit a member of staff who tried to tuck the bed sheet under the mattress.

Lucinda has now come in for another stay. On admission staff noticed immediately that Lucinda was walking very slowly and when sitting down she seemed to be very uncomfortable. The first night when a care assistant helps Lucinda undress she notices blood on her underwear. When questioned about this Lucinda say she has piles. Throughout this particular respite stay, Lucinda has been screaming out during the night but when staff have gone into her room they have found she is having nightmares. She has been screaming out 'Get him off me'; 'Stop it, I'm too old'. When questioned the next day, Lucinda says she doesn't remember dreaming.

Case Study 18

Subject: Gustav (age 85)

Gustav is a polish man who has lived in England for the past 60 years. He has never married and has always kept himself to himself. He had worked in a local factory since emigrating to England and although always amiable with his colleagues he did not mix with them socially outside of work. In his later years, he began having problems with arthritis and his mobility was reduced. A neighbour, Mrs Elliott, who is in her 70s, started coming in to visit him.

As Gustav's health deteriorated, the GP made a referral to social services for an assessment of need. Home carers were put in once a day for a morning call, in order to check on Gustav, get him up and dressed, light the fire and provide breakfast. Mrs Elliott said that she always visits at lunch time and provides something for him to eat; she also cashes his pension and ' buys him anything he needs'.

As they began to work with Gustav, the home carers found that he was always up when they arrived in the morning and was usually in the same clothes. They felt that he probably was sleeping downstairs and did not wash at all as he did smell and his skin was ingrained with dirt. He presented as very depressed and not being interested in anything. They are very concerned about the state of the house, which is very dirty, and the fact that there is hardly any food in the fridge. This morning they arrive to find there is no coal for the fire, no running water and the toilet is blocked.

Case Study 19

Subject: Emily (aged 90)

Emily had brought up her grandson, Grant, since he was a month old. Grant's mother (Emily's daughter) had run away and his father wanted nothing to do with him. Grant has always had a violent temper and in his teens he started getting into trouble with the police for fighting, shoplifting and stealing cars.

Grant is now 25 years old and still lives with his grandmother. He is unemployed and is always asking Emily for money. Emily has started attending a social services day centre two days a week and having some respite care. In recent months Emily has become very withdrawn and has been seen crying, but refuses to say what is upsetting her. She frequently comes to the day centre with no money and is very embarrassed when she cannot pay for her lunch.

Emily has now come in for a respite stay and she has two black eyes. She says she walked into a door. A new care assistant has begun work who knows Grant and Emily because she lives near them. She tells the manager of the home that Grant is a well-known drug dealer in the community.

Case Study 20

Subjects: Jessica (aged 90) and Harriet (aged 85)

Jessica and Harriet are sisters who have always lived together; neither of them have married and they have no other family. Harriet has been 'pleasantly confused' for years now, but Jessica had always managed to care for her with full support from home care services, day care and regular respite care. Jessica had a stroke six months ago which affected her left side. Both sisters were placed together permanently in an unfamiliar residential home, because there had been no vacancies in the home where Harriet had previously had day care and respite care.

Jessica is extremely unhappy with the care of her sister and has said to the manager, 'staff treat her like a child and we are not allowed to walk in the gardens outside the home'. Jessica herself hates being in the home because she feels 'It's like a prison. Meals are at set times and everyone has to be in bed by 10.30.' There are few residents she can have a conversation with and no activities available that interest her. She also resents having to pay staff to go to the shop and library for her as they will not accompany her because they 'haven't got the time to walk with a slow coach like you'.

Jessica does not know who to turn to for help. The social worker has not visited the sisters since the first review, which took place six weeks after they had been placed in the home.

Appendix

Suggested Reading

A growing amount of literature related to adult abuse has appeared in the last decade. Potential trainers may wish to undertake their own literature search, but many trainers (like those who are going to be part of a pool and already have full-time jobs) will have limited time to search, read and learn materials. The list presented below is limited. My aim is to present the potential trainer with materials that give him/her insight into the basics. They are also the materials that I personally have found most useful and I hope will point trainers in the right direction.

Adult abuse

Action on Elder Abuse (2000) *Training and Elder Abuse.* London: Action on Elder Abuse.

Aitken, L. and Griffin, G. (1996) *Gender Issues in Elder Abuse.* London: Sage.

ARC/NAPSAC (1993) *It Could Never Happen Here!: The Prevention and Treatment of Sexual Abuse with Learning Disabilities in Residential Settings.* Chesterfield and Nottingham: ARC/NAPSAC.

Biggs, S., Phillipson, C. and Kingston, P. (1995) *Elder Abuse in Perspective.* Buckingham: Open University Press.

Brown, H. (1999) *Aims for Adult Protection: The Alerter's Guide and Training Manual.* Brighton: Pavilion Publishing.

Brown, H. (1999) *Aims for Adult Protection: The Investigator's Guide and Training Manual.* Brighton: Pavilion Publishing.

Brown, H. (1994) ' Lost in the system: acknowledging the sexual abuse of adults with learning disabilities.' *Care in Place 9*, 2, 145–147.

Brown, H. and Stein, J. (1998) 'Implementing adult protection policies in Kent and East Sussex.' *Journal of Social Policy 27*, 3, 371–396.

Brown, H., Stein, J. and Turk, V. (1995) 'Report of a second two year incidence survey on the reported sexual abuse of adults with learning disabilities: 1991 and 1992.' *Mental Handicap Research 8*, 1, 1–22.

Clough, R. (ed) (1996) *The Abuse of Care in Residential Institutions.* London: Whiting and Birch.

Decalmer, P. and Glendenning, F. (eds) (1997) *The Mistreatment of Elderly People.* 2nd Edition. London: Sage.

Department of Health (1993) *No Longer Afraid: the safeguard of older people in domestic settings.* London: HMSO.

Department of Health (2000) *No Secrets: guidance on developing and implementing multi-agency policies and procedures to protect vulnerable adults from abuse.* London: HMSO.

Eastman, M. (1984) *Old Age Abuse.* London: Age Concern.

Eastman, M. (1994) *Old Age Abuse: A New Perspective.* London: Chapman and Hall.

Pritchard, J. (1995) *The Abuse of Older People.* 2nd Edition. London: Jessica Kingsley Publishers.

Pritchard, J. (1996) *Working with Elder Abuse: A Training Manual For Home Care, Residential And Day Care Staff.* London: Jessica Kingsley Publishers.

Pritchard, J. (ed) (1999) *Elder Abuse Work: Best Practice in Britain and Canada.* London: Jessica Kingsley Publishers.

Pritchard, J. (2000) *The Needs of Older Women: Services for Victims of Elder Abuse and Other Abuse.* Bristol: Policy Press.

Slater, P. and Eastman, M. (eds) (1999) *Elder Abuse: Critical Issues in Policy and Practice.* London: Age Concern.

Stanley, N., Manthorpe, J. and Penhale, B. (eds) (1999) *Institutional Abuse: Perspectives Across the Life Course.* London: Routledge.

Turk, V. and Brown, H. (1993) 'The sexual abuse of adults with learning disabilities: results of a two year incidence survey.' *Mental Handicap Research 6,* 3, 193–216.

Williams, C. (1995) *Invisible Victims: Crime and Abuse Against People with Learning Difficulties.* London: Jessica Kingsley Publishers.

Adult Learning

Ashworth, P. and Saxton, J. (1990) 'On "competence"'. *Journal of Further and Higher Education 14,* 2, 8–25

Cross, P. (1981) *Adults as learners.* San Francisco: Jossey-Bass.

Honey, P. and Mumford, A. (1982) *The Manual of Learning Styles.* Maidenhead: Honey.

Hyland, T. (1995) 'Behaviourism and the meaning of competence' in P. Hodkinson and M. Issitt (eds) *The Challenge of Competence.* London: Cassell.

Kolb, D.A. (1984) *Experiential Learning: Experience as the Source of Learning and Development.* New York: Prentice Hall.

NACRO Training and Development Services (1992) *A Guide to Good Practice in Training.* London: NACRO.

Schon, D.A. (1983) *The Reflective Practitioner.* London: Arena.

Schon, D.A. (1987) *Educating the Reflective Practitioner.* San Francisco: Jossey-Bass.

Yelloly, M. and Henkel, M. (1995) *Learning and Teaching in Social Work: Towards Reflective Practice.* London: Jessica Kingsley Publishers.

Evaluation of training

Bell, L. and Beard, A. (1996) *Get Going: A Guide to the Evaluation of Training.* Milton Keynes: Joint Initiative for Community Care.

Bramley, P. (1991) *Evaluating Training Effectiveness: Translating Theory Into Practice.* London: McGraw-Hill

Hamblin, A.C. (1974) *The Evaluation and Control of Training.* New York: McGraw-Hill.

Weiss, C.H. (1972) *Evaluation Research: Methods of Assessing Program Effectiveness.* Englewood Cliffs, NJ: Prentice Hall.

Legal matters

British Medical Association and Law Society. (1995) *Assessment of Mental Capacity: Guidance for Doctors and Lawyers.* London: British Medical Association Law Society.

Gunn, M.J. (1994) *Sex and the Law: A Brief Guide for Staff Working with People with Learning Difficulties.* London: Family Planning Association.

Home Office (1998) *Speaking Up For Justice.* London: HMSO.

Home Office (March 1999) *Action for Justice.* London: HMSO.

Lord Chancellor's Department (1997) *Who Decides? Making Decisions on Behalf of Mentally Incapacitated Adults.* London: The Stationery Office.

Useful journals

Journal of Adult Protection (Pavilion Publishing).

Journal of Elder Abuse and Neglect (USA).

Useful organisations

(for links to information, newsletters, publications, training materials)

Action on Elder Abuse, Astral House, 1268 London Road, London SW16 4ER.

Ann Craft Trust (ACT), Centre for Social Work, University of Nottingham, University Park, Nottingham, NG7 3RD.

British Institute of Learning Disabilities, Wolverhampton Road, Kidderminster, Worcestershire DY10 3PP.

Practitioner Alliance Against Abuse of Vulnerable Adults (PAVA),

P.O. Box 305, Barnsley S71 5YL.

UK Voice, P.O. Box 238, Derby DE1 9JN.

Index